Adapted Physical Education for Adults with Disabilities

3rd Edition

Peggy Lasko-McCarthey, Ph.D.

Karl G. Knopf, Ed.D.

eddie bowers publishing, inc.
2600 Jackson Street
Dubuque, IA 52001

eddie bowers publishing, inc.
2600 Jackson Street
Dubuque, Iowa 52001

ISBN 0-945483-13-9

Printed in the United States of America.

9 8 7 6 5 4 3 2

Contents

Preface

This instructional text was developed for the use of program directors, instructors, and assistants involved in adapted physical education programs for disabled adults. Very few comprehensive books exist on adapted physical education at the post-secondary level; even fewer materials exist on how to train assistants in these programs. Because the success of individualized exercise programs depend on the skills of assistants, thorough training is essential. It is the intent of this text to guide and supplement the instructor's efforts in this enormous task.

Gratitude is expressed to Sam Britten, Ph.D. (California State University, Northridge), Margie Corbett, and James Burke, M.A. (San Diego State University) for their extensive contributions in adapted exercise programs for adults with disabilities. A special thanks to James Burke who wrote Chapter 14 on "Sports Participation." We would like to acknowledge the following people for volunteering as models in the exercise photographs: Rick Lasko, Wendy Borgerd, and Dory Cox. Jennifer Quin and Michael Lung posed for the photograph on the cover.

We dedicate this text to our children, Alexandra McCarthey and Christopher and Kevin Knopf; to our supportive spouses, Eric McCarthey and Margaret Knopf; and in loving memory of Frank Parodi.

We express our heartfelt thanks to the many adults with disabilities who have participated in our programs over the years. They have provided the impetus for this text and have significantly influenced its contents. We sincerely hope that our adapted physical education programs have enriched their lives as much as it has ours.

Peggy Lasko-McCarthey, Ph.D.
Karl G. Knopf, Ed.D.

About the Authors

Peggy Lasko-McCarthey, Ph.D. was an assistant professor of adapted physical education and motor development at San Diego State University. She was the former Program Director of the Fitness Clinic for the Physically Disabled at San Diego State University from 1980-86. Dr. Lasko-McCarthey has lectured nationally and published articles regarding physical fitness for adults with disabilities. Her research focus is on developing graded exercise test protocols for persons with cervical spinal cord injuries.

Karl G. Knopf, Ed.D. is the Division Assistant of Special Education at Foothill College. Dr. Knopf has had extensive experience with physically challenged adults in the field of adapted physical education. He has published two additional books entitled *Water Workout* and *Fitness over Fifty*. He has served as a consultant to the California Community Colleges Chancellor's office on adapted physical education program evaluation and credentialing.

Developing an Adapted Physical Education Program for Adults with Disabilities

> *A teacher who makes little or no allowance*
> *for individual differences in the classroom*
> *is an individual who makes little or*
> *no difference in the lives of his/her students.*
>
> - William A. Ward

Introduction

Background and Scope of Post-Secondary, Adapted Physical Education Programs

Exercise has long been acknowledged as an essential component of the rehabilitation process for adults with disabilities; yet, in the past, many of those adults have typically failed to engage in regular physical activity *after discharge* from hospital-based therapy, due to the unavailability of college-based or community-based exercise programs. An encouraging development of recent years has been the realization that *continued* physical activity beyond the hospital can make a major contribution in the lives of persons with disabilities. Being physically competent enhances a person's self-image, confidence, and feelings of control, all of which are important to vocational, social, and intellectual growth. As Julian Stein stated in reference to persons with disabilities, "Give me pride; give me substance; give me a life of my own and I'll stop feeding off of yours." These beliefs have led to the growth of physical activity programs for adults at colleges (both two and four year), city recreation departments, YMCAs, and even hospitals.

Federal (Public Law 93-112) and state (in California, Assembly Bill 77) legislation have mandated the right of persons with disabilities to access physical education programs at the post-secondary level where similar programs exist for able-bodied persons. These laws have provided the impetus for post-secondary physical educators, adapted physical educators, and special educators to work together to assure quality physical education for adults with disabilities. The general theme of these laws is that physical education programs for persons with disabilities should be free, appropriate, and individualized. Because adaptations are often necessary in programs of this nature, the term adapted physical education (APE) is used at most colleges. Programs are typically sponsored by departments of physical education and/or on-campus disabled services. Undergraduate and graduate students in adapted physical education, sports medicine, and allied disciplines such as nursing generally receive college credit for assisting with individualized exercise programs. Participants with disabilities normally enroll in these classes through the regular registration process. If the program is conducted as an auxiliary program for non-students from the community, enrollment may be handled within the program itself and any fees charged to participants may be determined by the amount of financial support from the institution, grants, and local agencies.

Adapted physical education at the post-secondary level is defined as a diversified psychomotor and educational experience in which the teaching styles and activities are modified to insure success for each individual adult (Sherrill, 1986). Adapted physical education differs from regular physical education in that it features individualized programs of instruction. The scope of APE programs at the post-secondary level may vary from clinical habilitation and physical fitness programs to those that provide modified sports and recreation. The focus of a specific APE program will reflect the needs of the surrounding community and may include any combination of the following areas: muscular strength and endurance, cardiovascular endurance, flexibility, posture, static and dynamic balance, locomotion, perceptual-motor skills, sports-related gross motor skills, and fine motor skills. Whatever the focus, the APE program should be designed in conjunction with medical consultation and recommendations from each participant's physician. Many times adapted physical educators coordinate their programming efforts with those of physical therapists, occupational therapists, and kinesiotherapists to provide the most comprehensive and beneficial wellness plan for the participant. Where appropriate, opportunities should also be provided within the APE program for activities which develop social skills and self-esteem.

An important point to remember is that adapted physical educators work "with" and not "on" individuals with disabilities. This statement implies that the participant is involved with the adapted physical educator in the decision-making process every step of the way, from the establishment of exercise objectives to the evaluation of progress.

Participants involved in an APE program at the post-secondary level may have either congenital and acquired disabilities. Examples of the latter include such disabilities as cerebrovascular accident (i.e., stroke), traumatic spinal cord injury, visual impairment, acquired brain injury, and degenerative neuromuscular diseases, to name but a few. The individual with a recently acquired medical condition may still be adjusting to the disability, both physically and emotionally. Therefore, additional personnel such as a social worker or psychologist may provide pertinent information that will assist in determining the most appropriate teaching approach to utilize with the participant.

Unfortunately, research and dissemination of knowledge in APE at the post-secondary level has not kept pace with the growth of such programs. The intent of this manual is to provide program directors, instructors, and assistants guidance in establishing and executing post-secondary, APE programs for adults with disabilities. It is not possible to cover within this manual the entire scope of APE programs, particularly adapted sports. Therefore, the primary focus will be limited to chapters on muscular strength and endurance, flexibility, cardiovascular endurance, gait, perceptual-motor skills, posture, and adapted aquatics. Some brief information on wheelchair sports and goalball for persons with visual impairments is presented in Chapter 14.

Benefits of Adapted Physical Education Programs

The question of how exercise is beneficial to the person with a disability can best be explained by considering the deleterious effects of disuse syndrome. Disuse syndrome results from disruption of the normal balance between rest and physical activity, thereby decreasing the optimal functional capacity of an individual (Valbona, 1982). Inactivity due to immobilization (e.g., sitting or recumbent) reduces both the opportunity for active muscle contractions and the influence of gravity on weight-bearing bones. Depending on the organ or system involved, disuse syndrome can develop within as little as 3 days of immobilization (Talbot et al.; Valbona, 1982). Medical complications of disuse syndrome are numerous, producing the following physiologic and biochemical changes in organs and systems of the body (Valbona, 1982):

1. decreased physical work capacity
2. muscle atrophy
3. negative nitrogen and protein balance
4. osteoporosis
5. contracture of connective tissue
6. renal liathisis
7. cardiovascular deconditioning
8. pulmonary restrictions
9. decubiti ulcers
10. mental depression

Users of wheelchairs who are sedentary are especially prone to disuse syndrome and a lowered functional capacity. When disuse syndrome is coupled with a disability and aging, the result is more functional loss than would be predicted by the disability alone (Lasko-McCarthey & Aufsesser, 1990). The greater the loss in functional capacity, the greater the loss of independence in activities of daily living (unless the individual has access to technological advances which restore independence).

Exercise can prevent, minimize, or reverse the effects of disuse syndrome and should be available to all persons with disabilities, even if those disabilities are severe. Athough exercise may vary in type and mode, all forms of exercise provide some degree of mental and physical benefits for adults with disabilities, including the following (Lasko-McCarthey & Aufsesser, 1990; Pollock, Wilmore, & Fox, 1984):

1. Maintaining optimal health and decreasing the incidence of secondary health problems related to disuse syndrome.
2. Increasing muscular strength and endurance, resulting in less expenditure of energy to perform activities of daily living.
3. Increasing flexibility.
4. Improving cardiovascular function and blood lipid management.
5. Reducing risk factors responsible for cardiovascular disease.
6. Preventing obesity and glucose intolerance.
7. Preventing sport-related injuries.
8. Reducing mental stress.
9. Improving sleep.
10. Enhancing self-esteem and a feeling of control.
11. Improving basic motor skills which may allow an individual to develop prevocational or vocational skills.

How to Develop a Post-Secondary Adapted Physical Education Program

This next section provides guidelines for establishing a post-secondary APE program. In addition to these suggestions, recruitment of participants and assistants may be a necessary part of developing your program. Publicizing the program can be accomplished via brochures, video tape or slide show, presentations at agencies representing adults with disabilities, contacts with local therapists and physicians, and advertising through disabled services and the school newspaper.

Procedures for Program Admission

Before any physical assessment is conducted by the APE instructor, it is desirable for the potential participant to undergo a medical examination by a physician, noting any contraindications to exercise, including cardiopulmonary or orthopedic limitations, metabolic dysfunction, and medications (Hall, Meyer, & Hellerstein, 1984; Pollock, Wilmore, & Fox, 1978). The American College of Sports Medicine (ACSM) (1986) recommends that physically inactive persons over 35 years of age and persons of any age with coronary heart disease risk factors receive a medical examination before engaging in a regular program of exercise. Furthermore, ACSM recommends an exercise stress test prior to beginning an exercise program for healthy adults over the age of 45 years. The test should be performed in the presence of a physician. Graded exercse tests are important not only to confirm the safety of exercise but also to determine functional capacity which will serve as the basis for any cardiovascular exercise prescription.

Although these suggestions may seem burdensome to the participant, the more information known before training, the safer and more accurate the individualized exercise program will be.

All participants, regardless of age, should obtain a medical release from a personal physician prior to participation in the program. The illustration below shows a typical medical release form that may be sent to the physician. A general description of the APE program should be provided on the release form to orient the physician about the nature of the program. It is suggested that the following items be requested on the medical

Sample medical release form to be signed by a physician.

SAN DIEGO STATE UNIVERSITY
Department of Physical Education
Fitness Clinic for the Physically Disabled
MEDICAL RELEASE FORM

TO:
FROM: Peggy Lasko, Program Director
RE PATIENT:

This letter is to inform you that the above named individual has enrolled in the Fitness Clinic for the Physically Disabled at San Diego State University. This program involves individualized exercise programs (with or without assistance) for improvements in muscular strength, range of motion, cardiovascular endurance, posture, and balance. In order for the instructors to provide a safe and beneficial activity program, it is requested that you examine the individual to determine his/her eligibility to perform in the above named activity. It is also requested that you provide any medical information which would affect the selection of activities. Usually the case history with the physician's recommendations and limitations have been the most helpful with past programs. All medical records will be handled in strict confidence. Thank you for your cooperation.

Diagnosis: _____
_____

Resting blood pressure: _____
EXERCISE PROGRAM (Please check)
_____ No contraindications or restrictions requiring special instructions.
_____ Contraindicated activities (please list):

_____
_____

_____ Special exercise for:

_____
_____

Signed_____ , M.D.   Date _____
Type name here: _____   Phone _____
Address _____   Zip _____
        Street   City
Please return to: Peggy Lasko
        Department of Physical Education
        San Diego State University, San Diego, CA 92182-0171
I hereby authorize release of pertinent medical records to Peggy Lasko, Department of Physical Education, San Diego State University.

_____   _____
Signature of Patient   Date

Sample intake form to be filled out by the participant.

SAN DIEGO STATE UNIVERSITY
Department of Physical Education
Fitness Clinic for the Physically Disabled

MEDICAL HISTORY/HEALTH HABIT QUESTIONAIRE

<u>PART I</u> - PRESENT MEDICAL HISTORY

Date of Interview_____ Interviewer_____
Name_____ Age_____ Birthdate_____
Address_____ Zip Code_____
Phone Numbers: Day_____Evening_____
Soc. Sec. No. _____Vehicle Lic. No._____
Place of Birth _____
Height _____ Weight _____ Sex _____ Race_____
Resting Heart Rate_____ Resting Blood Pressure_____
In case of emergency contact:_____
Phone _____ Address_____

1. LIST ALL MEDICATIONS PRESENTLY TAKING

Medication   Dose   Purpose   Duration   Side Effects
_____
_____
_____
_____

2. MEDICAL DIAGNOSES: (include date of onset or occurance)
_____
_____
_____
_____

Page2

3. PRESENT MEDICAL CONDITION:
_____
_____
_____
_____

4. EXERCISE CONTRAINDICATIONS:
_____
_____

5. OPERATIONS (Since onset or occurrence of disability)

Type   Reason   Date   Complications
_____
_____
_____
_____

6. THERAPY RECEIVED DURING PAST YEAR:

Type   Reason   Duration   Where
_____
_____
_____

7. LIST YOUR PHYSICIANS

Name_____Specialty_____ Phone_____
Address_____ Zip _____
Frequency of visits_____ Reason_____
Name_____Specialty_____ Phone_____
Address_____ Zip _____
Frequency of visits_____ Reason_____

---

release: (1) medical diagnosis; (2) resting blood pressure; (3) exercise contraindications or restrictions; and (4) physician's recommendations for exercise. All of this information assists in planning a safe and beneficial program.

The instructor should additionally develop an intake form which includes: (1) general information regarding the participant (e.g., address, phone number); (2) a personal contact in case of emergency; (3) medications taken by the participant, including dose, frequency, and side effects; (4) medical history prior to and since onset of the disability; (5) pertinent operations; (6) whether participant is receiving any type of therapy; and (7) a list of the participant's physicians (see illustration on the left).

Physical Assessment

Physical assessment of the participant is essential because it provides the instructor with data to: (1) establish the participant's current level of performance; (2) identify realistic and individualized exercise goals; (3) prescribe appropriate, adapted exercises; and (4) monitor progress upon post-testing. The assessment should begin by jointly determining the participant's long and short term goals. Information provided on the medical release and intake forms, as well as the participant's goals, direct the type of assessment conducted by the instructor. Subsequent chapters in this manual describe the types of assessment the instructor may carry out, depending on the participant's needs. Sample assessment forms are also located in these chapters. Before beginning the assessment, the instructor should be familiar with contraindications to exercise testing and reasons for terminating an exercise test as outlined in Chapter 15. Post-testing is also recommended at the end of the program to determine whether the individual's program goals have been met.

Program Implementation

Once the medical history and release have been obtained and physical assessment completed, the task of individualized exercise programming may begin. Assessment data should be blended with the participant's medical history, type and severity of disability, age, personal long and short term goals, and physician's recommendations to produce an individualized exercise program. The participant's input should be considered essential to the development of this program. Input from other allied health professionals working with the participant may also be helpful in creating the optimal exercise program and teaching style. Periodic feedback from the participant and his/her assistant will insure that the exercise program is achieving the objectives set forth at the start of the program. Later chapters in this manual address guidelines for implementing specific portions of the APE program.

Record Keeping and the Exercise Program Card

It is *strongly* suggested that a file be kept on site for each participant. This file should contain all paperwork involved in program admission, physical assessment, and program implementation (e.g., medical history, medical release, assessment forms, completed exercise program cards). Ideally, the medical release should be updated each time the participant re-enrolls in the program. Any significant change in the participant's medical condition would also warrant an updated medical release from his/her physician. For liability purposes, the participant's file should be kept until the statute of limitation runs out on a person's right to litigate for negligence.

The instructor should write out each individual's entire exercise program on cards or paper that he/she can use to record information on daily. Some APE programs have stored their particpants' exercise programs in computer files, eliminating the laborious process of writing up programs. The exercise cards should contain the following information:

1. name of participant
2. dates for every day the participant exercised in the program
3. names of exercises, techniques and body positions used, and prescriptions
4. daily recording of quantitative data related to performance (e.g., number of sets, repetitions, and weight lifted for strength exercises; resting and exercising heart rates, resting and exercising blood pressures, duration of exercise, and work rates for cardiovascular training)
5. any exercise contraindications.

In addition, a card for "progress notes" can be attached to the exercise program card to allow for recording of qualitative information (e.g., pain occurring during an exercise bout; motivational level of participant). The assistant should never change the exercises on the program card without approval from the instructor. For liability purposes, the assistant should insure that the card is filled out completely and dated on a daily basis.

Consistent terminology should be used when describing exercises on the program card. This procedure allows for interchanging of assistants without confusion. Exercises can be named according to the following system:

1. **Anatomical movement:** For single joint movements, write the name of the joint and its anatomical movement. The body position will also have to be indicated. For example, "knee flexion - prone." All anatomical movements and body positions are described in Chapter 2.
2. **Approved vernacular:** If multi-joint movement is involved in performing the exercise, then use an approved vernacular that is understood by all in the program. For example, "lat pull" or "bench press."
3. **Abbreviated description:** If the exercise has been modified for an individual or there is no accepted name for it, a brief description should be written in.

The illustration on the next page is a sample exercise program card for a participant with an incomplete, cervical spinal cord injury.

Methods to Enhance Your Program Budget

If the exercise program budget is limited, there exist other avenues by which to acquire equipment and supplies. In fact, these avenues should always be explored to avoid any unnecessary purchases out of a limited program budget.

1. **Federal, state, and local grants.** Check both public (government) and private (foundations) grant opportunities. Most colleges house a grants office where you can obtain the names and addresses of federal, state, and local funding sources.
2. **Donations.** Mail letters to your local community organizations requesting equipment donations and/or money. Agencies which provide services to persons with disabilities may also provide money if their clients are enrolled in your program. Local businesses may be willing to donate items such as carpets and mirrors to your program.
3. **Homemade equipment.** An assistant may be able to build/sew certain pieces of equipment (e.g., treatment tables, balance boards, bean bags, quad gloves) at a dramatically reduced cost. A note of caution - because homemade equipment is not subject to any industry standards, liability for injury would befall the instructor. Therefore, homemade equipment should be rigorously inspected on a regular basis for any defects.
4. **Loan/sharing.** The physical education department within your college may be willing to loan or share a piece of equipment (i.e., assessment tools).
5. **Fundraisers** such as t-shirt sales (with program logo), bake sales, and wheel-a-thons.
6. **Use of community/private facilities.** Check in your local area on the availability of recreation centers, municipal pools, bowling alleys, and archery ranges.

Sample exercise cards for (a) arm cycle ergometry and (b) manually assisted exercises.

a ADAPTED PHYSICAL EDUCATION - EXERCISE PROGRAM

Name _____   Semester _____

EXERCISES:

ARM 1. Ergometer	Load / Time															
load (kp) time (min)	Load / Time															
	Load / Time															
	Load / Time															
Resting HR / Working HR																
Range for (.60-.80) Target HR = 114-152																

Pedal Rate = 60 rpm

b ADAPTED PHYSICAL EDUCATION- EXERCISE PROGRAM

Name _____   Semester _____

EXERCISES:

Active-assistive 10x 1. Dorsiflexion (longsit)															
Active-assistive 2. Hip flexion (supine-hook)															
Active 10x 3. Abdominal Curls (supine-hook)															
Active-assistive 10x 4. Hip abduction (side)															
Parallel bars:															
5. 4-point gait 10x															
6. Slide right and left 10x															
7. Standing balance 5x 10 sec. (arms abducted)															

Suggested Exercise Equipment

The equipment lists which follow are not meant to be inclusive but provide the basics for initiating an APE program. Because programs may vary dramatically in budget, facilities, and populations served, a universal equipment list does not exist. Due to the heterogeneous nature of participants served in these programs, equipment will be continually modified to meet the unique needs of individual adults. To keep updated on the latest equipment available, pick up vendors' catalogs in exhibitors' rooms at professional conferences (e.g., Annual Physical Activity Conference for the Exceptional Individual).

Considerable planning must precede the purchase of equipment for an APE program. The following is a list of factors to consider in the selection of exercise equipment.

1. The equipment should reflect the educational approach and objectives of the program. Is the program oriented towards developmental-habilitative activities, physical fitness, recreational/leisure activities, or adapted sports?
2. The instructor should consider what the future directions of the program are (i.e., can the equipment be modified later to accommodate changes?).
3. Is the equipment appropriate for the populations and ages served by the program?
4. Is the equipment appropriate for the developmental or skill level of the participants?
5. Is the exercise room large enough to house the equipment?
6. Is the equipment durable and washable?
7. Does the equipment have versatility?

Assessment Equipment

1. **Physician's weight scale.**
2. **Sitting weight scale** for wheelchair users.
3. **Posture screen or plumb line.** The design for construction of a homemade posture screen is located in Appendix C.
4. **Dynamometers.** These measure grip and pinch strength. More sensitive dynamometers are available (usually rubber bulbs which can be squeezed) to accommodate extreme paresis or contractures of the hand.
5. **Goniometers.** These devices measure range of motion about a joint.
6. **Skin fold calipers.** The Lange and Harpenden calipers are perhaps the most frequently used calipers and measure skin fold thickness at specified sites to calculate percent body fat.
7. **Ergometers** (arm and leg cycles). Cardiovascular endurance is measured by these devices. Monark, Bodyguard, and Fitron (Lumex) are popular brands that allow for precise testing.
8. **Metronome.** This device helps maintain the desired cadence (arm or leg) during ergometer tests.
9. **Stopwatches.** These are necessary for measuring time during testing and training, as well as for calculating resting and exercising heart rates.
10. **Sphygomometer (blood pressure cuff).** Resting and exercising blood pressures should always be taken during an ergometer test.

11. **Stethoscope.** This is used in conjunction with the blood pressure cuff.
12. **Orthotron or Cybex (Lumex).** Both dynamometers are used in assessing isokinetic strength in major joints of the body. The former is considerably less expensive than the latter but is less precise in measurement and less sensitive. Both devices are utilized for training purposes as well.
13. **Spirometer.** Lung volumes and flow rates are measured with this device. The values obtained are usually greatly reduced in respiratory conditions and when paralysis of the trunk muscles has occurred.
13. **Anthropometric tape.** Limb circumferences are measured with this special tape to determine any muscular atrophy.
14. **Sit and reach box.** This apparatus measures the flexibility of the hamstrings and low back muscles. See Appendix D for the construction of a homemade box.

Equipment for Developing Strength and Range of Motion

1. **Sliding board.** This board is used in supine and side-lying positions for movements performed actively (e.g., hip flexion and abduction). Covering the surface with linoleum or talc reduces friction (and thus resistance) created by the limb against the board. This term also refers to a beveled, rectangular board used for transferring an individual from a wheelchair to another surface of equal height.
2. **Ankle boot.** Used for strengthening the ankle.
3. **Push-up blocks.** Used for strengthening the shoulder and elbow muscles involved in transfers.
4. **Overhead pulley with swivel hook.** This self-assistive device is used for range of motion of the shoulder joints.
5. **Standing frame.** Enables non-ambulatory persons an opportunity to stand supported at the waist and knees.
6. **Light dumbbells and/or ankle and wrist weights.** Use one-half to one pound increments up to 10 pounds; use five to ten pound increments thereafter.
7. **Kinetron (Lumex).** This isokinetic device is used for developing strength and coordination of the leg muscles involved in walking.
8. **Shoulder wheel.** Improves range of motion at the shoulder joint.
9. **Freedom Machine (Olympic Enterprises).** This four-sided machine was designed to strengthen the upper extremities of wheelchair users. Several other similar devices are now available such the Equalizer 1000 (Helm Distributing). Stations typically include a vertical bench press, seated military press, rowing, high/low pulleys, lat pull down, vertical butterfly or peck-deck.
10. **Parallel bars and ambulation stairs.**
11. **Vinyl mats or low treatment tables.** Use 1" thickness for individual floor mats and low treatment tables and 2" mats for hazardous areas.
12. **Quad gloves.** These leather or vinyl gloves are used by persons with limited grip to secure dumbells, pulleys, or arm cycles to the hand (see Appendix E for a homemade pattern).
13. **Low and high plinths.** The bench surface should consist of 3/4 inch ply, padded with 2 inch vinyl covered foam. A modified bench for persons with

low extremity paralysis is designed with a narrow end that supports the head and shoulders but permits some mobility. A wide midsection and base stabilizes the trunk and provides support for transfers. Seat belts should be attached to provide lateral stability. This bench can then be situated under a wall pulley bar for upper extremity exercises.

14. **Universal Centurion Multi-station gym.**
15. **Universal leg extension/flexion gym.**
16. **Rickshaw exerciser.** This device is designed to strengthen muscles for wheelchair pushing and gait training.
17. **Theraplast.** This putty-like substance is used for grip and pinch strength.
18. **Adjustable chin-up bar** for supine position.
19. **Wall pulleys.** An entire bilateral strengthening routine for the upper extremities can be performed with this device.
20. **Wrist and ankle cuffs.** These leather cuffs can be attached to wall pulleys or lat pull machine by "S" hooks.
21. **Latex rubber tubing or bands.**
22. **Quad board.** This board is used for post-op knee rehabilitation and other conditions where knee flexion is restricted.

Equipment for Developing Cardiovascular Endurance

1. **Monark Rehab Trainer** (friction-braked arm ergometer).
2. **Friction-braked leg ergometers.**
3. **Rowcycle** (mobile) or stationary rowing machine.
4. **Wheelchair ergometer** (interfaced with friction-braked leg ergometer).
5. **Jump ropes.**

Perceptual-Motor Equipment

1. **Balls:** nerf, balloons, beach, cage (canvas), wiffle, medicine and rubber.
2. **Balance beams.** Widths: 2", 4", 6"
3. **Tilt boards.**
4. **Jump ropes.**
5. **Bean bags.**

Equipment for an Adapted Swim Program

1. **Portable Hoyer Lift.**
2. **Swim fins.**
3. **Snorkles.**
4. **Life vests** (small, medium, large).
5. **Kick boards.**
6. **Non-skid decking.**
7. **Rubber balls.**
8. **Donut inner tubes.**
9. **Hand paddles** (for persons with paraplegia and quadriplegia).
10. **Swim masks.**
11. **Floating basketball hoop and basketball.**

Miscellaneous Equipment

1. **Towels.** Participants should place a towel under their heads when lying on mats. This procedure reduces the need to frequently clean the mats, prevents the spread of illnesses, and minimizes allergic reactions to mold and dust.
2. **Stall bars.** These are used for a variety of activities such as range of motion and climbing.
3. **Masking/athletic tape.**
4. **Ace wraps** with 2", 4", 6", and 8" widths. The wraps are used for a variety of reasons, including the binding of hands to the pedals of arm cycle ergometers.
5. **Chalk board.**
6. **Walking belts** (small, medium, large). These facilitate transfers and reduce the chance of falling during parallel bars activities.
7. **Mirrors.** These are helpful with individuals who lack proprioception/body awareness.
8. **Storage cabinets.**
9. **First aid kit,** including instant cold packs.
10. **Laundry hamper** for towels.
11. **Bulletin board.**
12. **Velcro tape.**
13. **Seat belts** for securing participants into various exercise devices.
14. **Styrofoam cups** for drinking and making ice cups for first aid.
15. **Refrigerator or ice machine.** Ice is then available for first aid.
16. **Drinking straws** for water breaks.
17. **Spare wheelchair.**
18. **Spare crutches.**
19. **Fans** to combat hot weather.
20. **Disinfectant** to clean mats.
21. **Cleaning rags.**
22. **Broom and dust pan.**

Program Evaluation

To provide an objective yearly evaluation of the APE program, establish both community and medical advisory boards. Feedback from these groups can be obtained at the end of each academic year. The community advisory board may be composed of participants in the program, their family members, and representatives from allied local agencies (e.g., Multiple Sclerosis Society). The medical advisory board may be composed of physicians from various specialties (e.g., physical medicine, neurology, cardiology, and orthopedics) and therapists (e.g., physical, occupational, kinesiotherapy, recreational) who have referred participants to the APE program. These advisory boards can meet to review policies, operating procedures, number of participants, instructor to participant ratios, recruitment of future participants, and program fees. These boards may also assist in fund raising for the program and even help recruit volunteers to act as assistants.

Training Assistants

The success and efficiency of an APE program for adults with disabilities depends to a large extent upon how well assistants are trained. Large APE programs may offer introductory APE courses for assistants. These courses generally include didactic material and practical application. Smaller programs may not have this luxury and should schedule orientation sessions for assistants prior to the first day of the program. A training manual and/or video tapes are useful supplements to the orientation and reinforce concepts taught to assistants. To initiate the orientation, send a letter to all prospective assistants regarding the orientation schedule and the materials to be covered. A sample content of the orientation sessions is provided below:

1. Professional conduct, including use of appropriate language (see next section).
2. Grading and expectations.
3. Instructional strategies.
4. Emergency procedures during program operation.
5. General program procedures.
6. Assistant duties.
7. Equipment use and care.
8. Exercise techniques for developing strength, cardiovascular endurance, flexibility, balance, posture, and gait.
9. Review of files and medical histories of participants.
10. Information about specific disabilities.
11. Practice sessions.

Several orientation sessions may be required to cover all of the material presented above. It is suggested that each session last no more than three hours in duration. Allow assistants sufficient time to practice techniques acquired in the sessions. Using a competency checklist allows the instructor to screen assistants before assigning them to participants. In addition to the orientation, it is suggested that an open house be scheduled prior to the program to allow the potential participants to view the facility and meet the assistants.

Labels and Changing Attitudes Toward Persons with Disabilities

As one person with a disability said, "I can think of ways to deal with architectural barriers but attitudinal barriers are far more difficult." Attitudes towards persons with disabilities are often reflected in the labels used to identify and group them. Medical labels do have some benefit by providing legislators with rational for funding special education programs and services. However, incorrect or improper use of labels can inflict stigmatization and result in segration of individuals or groups. Stigmatization is the perception that a person is inferior because of differences associated with his/her disability. Unfortunately, stigmatization may generate sympathy or fear towards persons with disabilities, neither of which is desirable.

Another problem with labels that tend to segregate people is the phenomenon of stereotyping - associating particular characteristics to an entire group of persons and ignoring individuality. Stigmatization and stereotyping may lead to prejudice and discrimination in social, educational, and vocational settings. Thus, persons with disabilities are often externally limited much more by society's attitude regarding the disability than the actual disability itself. In addition, internal limits are created when the individual's perceptions of his/her ability are influenced by the negative views of others (French, Mastro, & Jackson, 1988). The familiar social-psychological axiom states that, "What you think of me, I will think of me, and what I think of me I will believe."

Two terms that influence attitudes and therefore warrant differentiation from each other are *handicap* and *disability*. These two terms are not synonymous. *Handicap* is generally defined as anything that prevents the attainment of one's goals (Sherrill, 1986). A person is *handicapped* if he/she encounters impediments or disadvantages that limit success in a given situation. Thus, being *handicapped* is situation specific; i.e., a person may be *handicapped* in one situation but not in others. In contrast, the term *disability* refers to the presence of a medical condition. For example, a person may have a *disability* because of a spinal cord injury to the thoracic vertebra, leaving him disabled or paralyzed in the leg muscles. This person is *handicapped* in regards to climbing stairs, but *only* if an elevator is not available. If an elevator is provided, then no *handicap* exists because the individual is able to accomplish his objective of getting to the second floor. This same person may not be *handicapped* at all in regards to archery, because his upper body strength was not affected by *disability*. Unfortunately, the word *handicapped* is still used interchangeably with *disability* in many legislative, educational, and administrative circles. Even federal legislation (e.g., Public Law 93-112, Public Law 94-142) have utilized the words *handicapped* and *disabled* synonymously.

In conclusion, instructors and assistants who work in APE programs must remember that the participants are individuals first and disabled second. For example, it is less desirable (from the participant's viewpoint) to use the term "epileptic" than the phrase, "person with epilepsy." The former defines the person in terms of his/her limitations while the latter places individuality first. Taken as a total human being, it is valid to assume that a person with a disability can do more than he/she cannot. Acceptable terminology will continue to change as a group's image changes. Two examples of phrases currently in vogue in reference to persons with physical disabilities are "physically challenged" and "differently abled." The bottom line is to be sensitive to word choices used in reference to persons with disabilities. Inappropriate word choices that have negative connotations include cripple, victim, invalid, patient (outside of a medical setting), abnormal, wheelchair bound or confined, and gimp. Again, these words have negative connotations because they define the individual in reference to his/ her limitations.

Intervention techniques to improve attitudes (French et al., 1988)

Below is a list of suggested activities designed to promote a better understanding of and empathy toward persons with disabilities, therefore improving attitudes.

1. Allow opportunities for assistants to observe how assistive devices are used by persons with disabilities. Have assistants experiment with ambulation aids (e.g., wheelchair, walker, crutches, cane). *Note* - emphasize to assistants that they should never take the liberty of sitting in an unoccupied wheelchair or "fooling around" with any device without the permission of the owner. These pieces of equipment should be considered intimate personal property and treated accordingly.

2. Encourage assistants to engage in an activity (e.g., lunch, tennis) with a person who is disabled.

3. Invite an athlete who is disabled to speak to the group of assistants about wheelchair sports.

4. Teach assistants the appropriate terminology in reference to persons with disabilities. The rule of thumb is to place the person before the disability.

5. Assign assistants and participants to observe a sporting event involving athletes with disabilities. Sports participation demonstrates ability, and whether integrated or segrated, can change how able-bodied persons view those with disabilities and how those with disabilities view themselves.

6. Encourage assistants to ask questions. Provide a mini-library of information for assistants to check-out overnight. In many cases, agencies that represent persons with disabilities will mail, free of charge, a packet of literature regarding the disability (e.g., Muscular Dystrophy Association, Multiple Sclerosis Society). These packets can be placed in folders and serve as the basis for the mini-library.

7. Simulate a disabling condition. For example, have assistants use their non-dominant hand to carry out activities of daily living; attempt to play a game such as tennis from a wheelchair; place plastic wrap over eyes to simulate a visual impairment. Discuss the difficulties encountered.

Study Questions / Learning Activities

1. List the benefits of regular physical exercise for persons with disabilities.

2. Identify the scope of post-secondary adapted physical education programs.

3. Outline the procedures involved in developing an individualized exercise program at the post-secondary level.

4. If you became permanently physically disabled, would any changes occur in your career choices, hobbies, friends, and method of learning in school? Answer the same question but substitute mental, learning, visual, and auditory disabilities for physical disabilities.

5. How can sports help to change stigmatization, stereotyping, and prejudice towards persons with disabilities?

6. Differentiate between the terms "disability" and "handicap". Provide an example to illustrate this difference.

7. What negative connotations does the word "handicapped" imply?

8. Develop two intervention techniques to improve your peer group's attitude toward persons with disabilities.

References

American College of Sports Medicine. (1986, 3rd ed.). *Guidelines for exercise testing and prescription*. Philadelphia: Lea & Febiger.

French, R., Mastro, J., & Jackson, S. (1988). Changing attitudes toward physically disabled: What can we do? *Clinical Kinesiology, 42*(3), 79-81.

Hall, L. K., Meyer, G. C., & Hellerstein, H. K. (1984). Cardiac rehabilitation: Exercise testing and prescription. New York: Spectrum Publications.

Lasko-McCarthey, P., & Aufsesser, P. M. (1990). Guidelines for a community-based physical fitness program for adults with physical disabilities. *Palaestra, 6*(4), 18-29.

Pollock, M., Wilmore, J., & Fox, S. (1984). *Exercise in health and disease*. Philadelphia: W. B. Saunders.

Sherrill, C. (1986). *Adapted physical education and recreation. A multidisciplinary approach*. Dubuque: William C. Brown.

Talbot, D., Pearson, V., & Loeper, J. (1978). *Disuse syndrome: The preventable disability*. Minneapolis: Sister Kennedy Institute.

Valbona, C. (1982, 3rd ed.). Bodily responses to immobilization. In: Kottke F. J., Stillwell G. K., Lehman J. F., eds. *Krusen handbook of physical medicine and rehabilitation*. Philadelphia: W. B. Saunders, pp. 963-75.

2

Basics in Anatomic Kinesiology

Critical to the development and implementation of individualized exercise programs is a basic understanding of anatomic kinesiology. This chapter will provide a foundation for those who have never taken a course in anatomic kinesiology and serve as a refresher for those who have.

Anatomical Directions

1. **Anterior/ventral**: Towards the front of the body.
2. **Posterior/dorsal**: Towards the back of the body.
3. **Superior/cranial/ cephalic/rostral**: Toward the head; one body part above another.
4. **Inferior/caudal**: Toward the feet; one body part below another.
5. **Medial**: Toward the midline of the body.
6. **Lateral**: Away from the midline of the body.
7. **Proximal**: A position nearest the source or midline.
8. **Distal**: A position farthest from the source.

Anatomical frames of reference. Subject is in anatomical position.

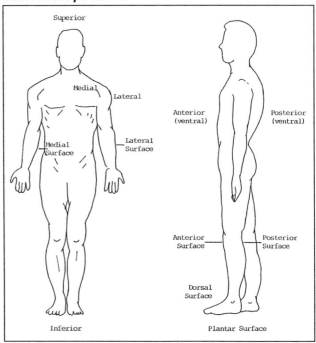

Anatomical Planes of the Body

Sagittal Plane

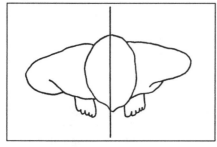

Sagittal Plane

Definition: The sagittal plane passes through the body from front to back, dividing the body into right and left segments.

Anatomical Movements:
1. flexion
2. extension
3. hyperextension

Frontal Plane

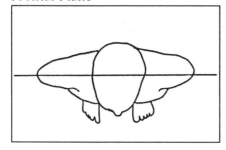

Frontal Plane

Definition: The frontal plane passes through the body laterally (from side to side), dividing it into anterior (front) and posterior (back) segments. Movement of the limbs must be toward or away from the midline of the body. The spine can flex to the right or left side.

Anatomical Movements:
1. abduction
2. adduction
3. lateral flexion

Transverse Plane

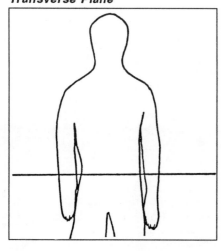

Transverse Plane

Definition: The transverse plane passes through the body horizontally, dividing it into superior (upper) and inferior (lower) segments. The spine can be rotated to the right or left, and the limbs can be rotated clockwise or counterclockwise from the midline of the body.

Anatomical Movements:
1. external (or outward) rotation
2. internal (or medial) rotation
3. supination
4. pronation
5. eversion
6. inversion
7. rotation right or left of the spine

Anatomical Movements

Anatomical movements are always described in reference to the "anatomical position." In this position, the individual stands erect, feet together, with the arms at the sides and palms facing forward. General anatomical movements are defined below.

General Anatomical Movements

Abduction - Movement away from the midline of the body in the frontal plane.

Adduction - Movement toward or beyond the midline of the body in the frontal plane.

Anterior Tilt - Forward tilt of the pelvic girdle (present in lordosis).

Circumduction - Movement circumscribing a conical area (e.g., hip and shoulder), involving flexion, abduction, extension, and adduction in sequence.

Depression - Downward movement of a part (e.g., shoulder and pelvic girdles).

Dorsiflexion - Flexion of the foot (ankle joint) upward.

Downward rotation - Movement of scapula as the arms are lowered. Superior border of the scapula moves away from the spine. Rotation of the scapula clockwise.

Elevation - Upward movement of a part (e.g., shoulder and pelvic girdles).

Eversion - Raising the lateral border of the foot.

Extension - Movement resulting in the increase of a joint angle (i.e., straightening at a joint). Return from flexion to anatomical position.

External (outward) rotation - Rotation of a bone in a clockwise direction away from the midline.

Flexion - Movement resulting in a decrease of a joint angle (i.e., bending at a joint).

Horizontal Abduction - With the shoulders flexed at 90 degrees (elbows extended), the arms move horizontally to the side of the body.

Horizontal Adduction - With the shoulders abducted at 90 degrees (elbows extended), the arms move horizontally to the front of the body.

Hyperextension - Movement beyond the position of extension.

Internal (medial) Rotation - Rotation of a bone in counterclockwise direction toward the midline.

Inversion - Raising the medial border of the foot up.

Lateral Flexion - Flexing the trunk or the neck to the left or the right in the frontal plane.

Plantar Flexion - Pointing or extending the foot (ankle joint) downward.

Posterior Tilt - Backward tilt of the pelvis.

Pronation - Foot: eversion combined with abduction of the forefoot. Forearm: rotating wrist or hand medially from elbow.

Protraction - Forward movement of a part (e.g., shoulder girdle).

Radial Deviation - Movement of the wrist and hand toward the radius.

Retraction - Backward movement of a part (e.g., shoulder girdle).

Rotation - Movement of a bone about its long axis.

Supination - Foot: inversion combined with adduction of the forefoot. Forearm: rotating wrist or hand laterally from elbow.

Ulnar Deviation - Movement of the wrist and hand toward the ulna.

Upward rotation - Movement of the scapula as the arms are raised. Superior border of the scapula moves toward the spine. Rotation of the scapula counterclockwise.

Specific joint movements are illustrated in the diagrams on pages 22-25.

Cervical Spine - Neck

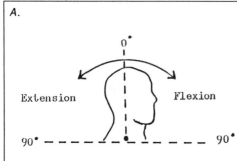

Cervical Spine - Neck

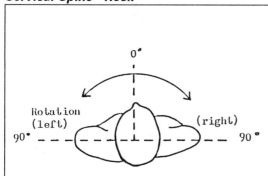

Shoulder Girdle

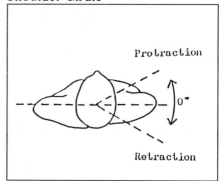

Shoulder Girdle

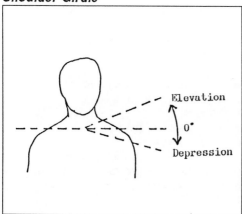

Shoulder

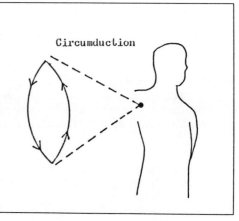

Shoulder

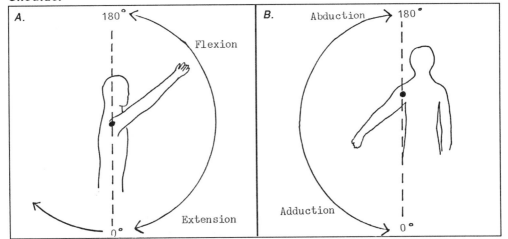

Shoulder

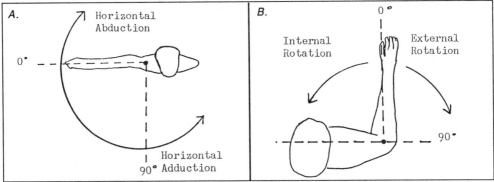

Elbow

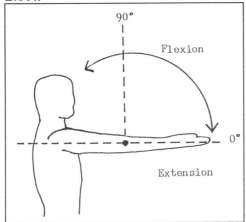

Forearm

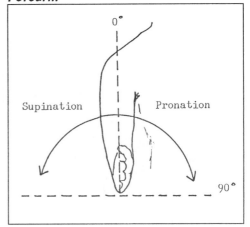

Spine

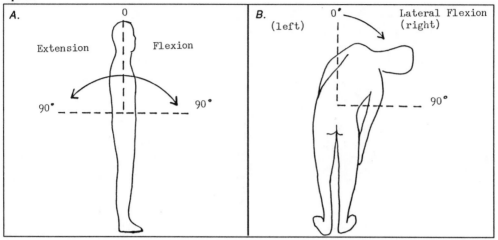

A.

Extension   0   Flexion

90°   90°

B.   0°   Lateral Flexion (right)

(left)

90°

Hip

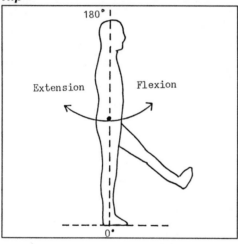

180°

Extension   Flexion

0°

Hip

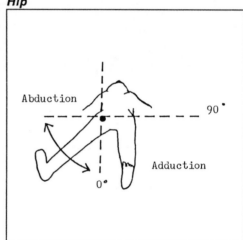

Abduction   90°

Adduction

0°

Hip

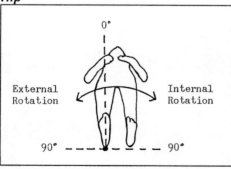

0°

External Rotation   Internal Rotation

90°   90°

Wrist

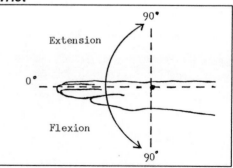

90°

Extension

0°

Flexion

90°

Knee

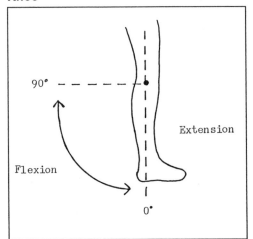

Ankle

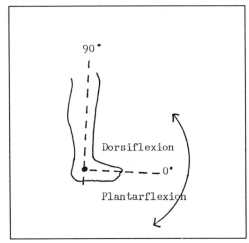

Ankle

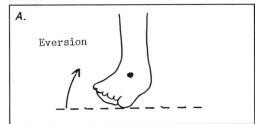

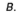

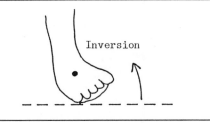

*(redrawn from **Joint motion**. American Academy of Orthopedic Surgeons, Chicago, 1965.)*

Short Hand for Anatomical Movements

Name	Short Hand	Name	Short Hand
Abduction	→	Hyperextension	H／
Adduction	←	Internal rotation	→ ◯◯◯◯
Flexion	∨	External rotation	← ◯◯◯
Extension	／		

Body Positions

Individualized exercise program cards should contain standard terminology whenever possible to avoid confusion when interchanging assistants with participants. The following illustrations on pages 26 and 27 show initial body positions for exercises and usually the associated terminology must be specified on the program card.

Cross Sitting

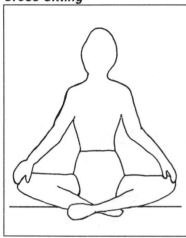

4-Point (all four extremities)

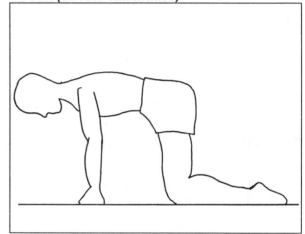

Long Sitting

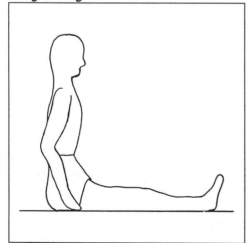

Hook Sitting

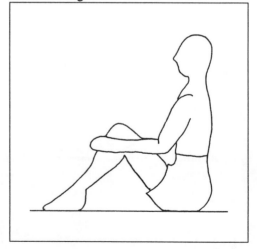

Hook Lying

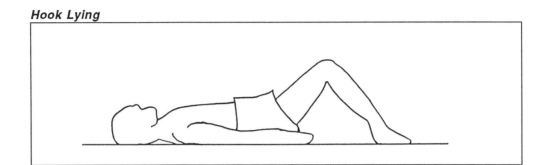

Supine

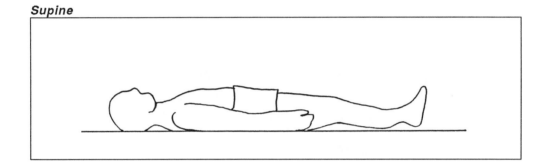

Side Lying

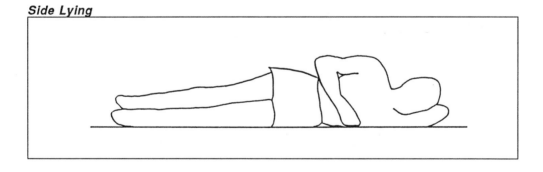

Prone

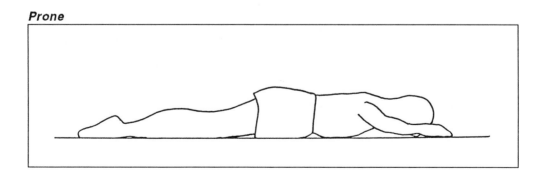

Muscles

Definition

A muscle is a bundle of contractile fibers held together by a sheath of connective tissue and attached to bone by means of a tendon. A muscle can be stretched and then returned to its normal resting length. Therefore, it is commonly said that muscles have extensibility and elastic properties. Muscles also have the capability to contract and develop tension because they respond to irritability and conductivity. It must be remembered that muscles are a neuromuscular unit and that without neurological innervation, movement cannot occur and atrophy will follow.

Muscles get their names for various reasons, including:

1. Action of the muscle (e.g., adductor longus)
2. Direction of fibers (e.g., transverse abdominus)
3. Location of the muscle (e.g., anterior tibialis)
4. Number of divisions comprising a muscle (e.g., biceps, triceps)
5. Shape of the muscle (e.g., trapezius, quadratus)
6. Point of attachment (e.g., sternocleidomastoid)

Roles in Which Muscle May Respond

Muscles can function in solo or as a member of a team. The following terms are used to desrcribe the various roles a muscle can assume.

- **Mover/Agonist**: Is the muscle responsible for concentric contractions. Mover/Agonist muscles are often subclassified as prime movers, or as assistant or secondary movers for a given action.
- **Prime Mover:** Is the muscle primarily responsible for eliciting a specific joint action.
- **Assistant Mover:** Is the muscle which aids the prime mover to effect a joint movement.
- **Antagonist:** Is a muscle that produces an action which is exactly the opposite of an agonist. An example of an antagonist is the biceps brachii, with respect to elbow extension (triceps brachii is the prime mover or agonist). For elbow flexion, the triceps brachii is the antagonist, while the biceps brachii is the prime mover.
- **Fixator/Stabilizer:** Is the muscle which anchors, steadies or supports a bone or body part to enable another muscle to have a firm base upon which to pull.
- **Synergist:** Is the muscle which acts along with some other muscle(s) as part of a team.
- **Neutralizer:** Is the muscle which contracts in order to counteract or neutralize an undesired action of another muscle which is acting upon that joint. This term is probably better than helping synergist or true synergist, because it avoids the various meanings attached to "synergist".

Types of Muscular Contractions

In kinesiology, the term "contraction" refers to the development of tension within a muscle. It does not imply that any shortening of muscle or movement has occurred at the joint.

- **Static/Isometric Contraction**: Occurs when muscle tension is equal to the resistance applied (e.g., gravity or an external load), preventing any movement; thus, the length of the muscle remains unchanged. Technically, no internal shortening of the contractile components occur because the muscle remains at the same length (i.e., statically contracted).

- **Concentric Contraction**: Occurs when a muscle develops sufficient tension to overcome a resistance (e.g., gravity or an external load), resulting in visible movement and shortening of the muscle (e.g., bringing your hand to your face is an example of a concentric contraction of the biceps brachii).

- **Eccentric Contraction**: Occurs when a resistance overcomes a contracting muscle so that the muscle actually lengthens without relaxing.

Muscles Involved in Anatomical Movement

Prime Movers (▼)   Assistant Movers (★)
(Nerve root level is indicated in parentheses)

Scapula

Elevation (C-1 to -5)
▼   Trapezius I & II
▼   Levator Scapulae
▼   Rhomboids

Upward Rotation (C-2 to C-8)
▼   Serratus Anterior
▼   Trapezius

Depression (C-4 to T-1)
▼   Trapezius IV
▼   Pectoralis Minor
★   Latissimus Dorsi

Downward Rotation (C-3 to T-1)
▼   Rhomboids
▼   Pectoralis Minor
★   Levator Scapulae

Glenohumeral Joint (shoulder)

Flexion (C-5 to T-1)
▼   Anterior Deltoid
▼   Pectoralis Minor
★   Biceps Brachii
★   Coracobrachialis

Abduction (C-5 to T-1)
▼   Middle Deltoid
▼   Supraspinatus
★   Anterior Deltoid
★   Triceps Brachii

Internal Rotation (C-5 to T-1)
▼   Subscapularis
▼   Teres Major
★   Anterior Deltoid
★   Pectoralis Minor
★   Biceps Brachii

Horizontal Adduction (C-5 to T-1)
▼   Anterior Deltoid
▼   Pectoralis Major
▼   Pectoralis Minor
▼   Coracobrachialis
★   Biceps Brachii

Extension (C-5 to T-1)
▼   Latissimus Dorsi
▼   Teres Major
★   Triceps Brachii
★   Posterior Deltoid

Adduction (C-5 to T-1)
▼   Pectoralis Major
▼   Latissimus Dorsi
▼   Teres Major
★   Biceps Brachii - short head
★   Triceps Brachii - short head

External Rotation (C-4 to C-6)
▼   Infraspinatus
▼   Teres Minor
★   Posterior Deltoid

Horizontal Abduction (C-4 to C-8)
▼   Middle Deltoid
▼   Posterior Deltoid
▼   Infraspinatus
▼   Teres Minor
★   Latissimus Dorsi
★   Teres Major

Ginglymus Joint (elbow)

Flexion (C-5 to T-1)
▼   Biceps Brachii
▼   Brachialis
▼   Brachioradialis
★   Flexor Carpi Radialis
★   Flexor Carpi Ulnaris

Extension (C-6 to T-1)
▼   Triceps Brachii
★   Anconeus
★   Extensor Carpi Radialis
★   Extensor Carpi Radialis Brevis
★   Extensor Carpi Ulnaris

Ginglymus Joint (elbow) - continued

Pronation (C-6 to T-1)
▼   Pronator Quadratus
★   Flexor Carpi Radialis
★   Pronator Teres

Supination (C-5 to T-1)
▼   Supinator
★   Extensor Carpi Radialis Longus
★   Extensor Pollicis Longus
★   Adductor Pollicis Longus
★   Biceps Brachii

Radiocarpal Joint (wrist)

Flexion (C-7 to T-1)
▼   Flexor Carpi Radialis
▼   Flexor Carpi Ulnaris
★   Palmaris Longus
★   Flexor Digitorum Profundus
★   Flexor Digitorum Superficialis
★   Extensor Indicis
★   Extensor Digii Minimi

Extension (C-6 to C-7)
▼   Extensor Carpi Radialis Longus
▼   Extensor Carpi Radialis Brevis
▼   Extensor Carpi Ulnaris
★   Extensor Digitorum

Trunk

Spinal Flexion (T-5 to T-12)
▼   Rectus Abdominis
★   Transversus Abdominis
★   External/Internal Obliques

Spinal Extension
▼   Sacrospinalis (Erector Spinae)

Hip Joint

Flexion (L-1 to S-3)
▼   Iliopsoas
▼   Rectus Femoris
▼   Pectineus
★   Tensor Fascia Latae
★   Gracilis
★   Adductor Longus
★   Adductor Magnus

Extension (L-4 to S-3)
▼   Gluteus Maximus
▼   Biceps Femoris
▼   Semitendinosus
▼   Semimembranosus
★   Gluteus Medius
★   Gluteus Minimus

Abduction (L-4 to S-1)
▼   Gluteus Medius
★   Iliopsoas
★   Sartorius
★   Rectus Femoris
★   Tensor Fasciae Latae
★   Gluteus Minimus

Adduction (L-1 to S-4)
▼   Pectineus
▼   Gracilis
▼   Adductor Longus
▼   Adductor Brevis
▼   Adductor Magnus

Internal Rotation (L-4 to S-2)
▼   Gluteus Minimus
★   Tensor Fasciae Latae
★   Semitendinosus
★   Semimembranosus
★   Muscles listed under adduction

External Rotation (L-1 to S-3)
▼   Gluteus Maximus
★   Sartorius
★   Iliopsoas
★   Biceps Femoris
★   Six external rotators are also assisting

Knee Joint

Flexion (L-2 to S-3)
- ▼ Semitendinosus
- ▼ Semimembranosus
- ▼ Biceps Femoris
- ★ Sartorius
- ★ Gracilis
- ★ Gastrocnemius
- ★ Plantaris

Extension (L-2 to L-4)
- ▼ Rectus Femoris
- ▼ Vastus Lateralis
- ▼ Vastus Intermedius
- ▼ Vastus Medialis

Internal Rotation (L-2 to S-5)
- ▼ Semitendinosus
- ▼ Semimembranosus
- ★ Sartorius
- ★ Gracilis
- ★ Popliteus

External Rotation (L-5 to S-3)
- ★ Biceps Femoris

Talocrural Joint (ankle)

Dorsiflexion (L-4 to S-1)
- ▼ Tibialis Anterior
- ▼ Extensor Digitorum Longus
- ★ Peroneus Tertius
- ★ Extensor Hallucis Longus

Plantarflexion (L-4 to S-2)
- ▼ Gastrocnemius
- ▼ Soleus
- ★ Plantaris
- ★ Peroneus Longus
- ★ Flexor Digitorum Longus
- ★ Flexor Hallucis Longus
- ★ Tibialis Posterior

Inversion (L-4 to L-5)
- ▼ Tibialis Anterior
- ▼ Tibialis Posterior
- ★ Flexor Digitorum Longus
- ★ Flexor Hallucis Longus
- ★ Extensor Hallucis Longus

Eversion (L-4 to S-1)
- ▼ Extensor Digitorum Longus
- ▼ Peroneus Tertius
- ▼ Peroneus Longus
- ▼ Peroneus Brevis

Respiratory Muscles

Inspiration (resting)
- ▼ Diaphragm
- ▼ External Intercostals
- ▼ Internal Intercostals
- ★ Erector Spinae

Inspiration (forced)
- ▼ Diaphragm
- ▼ External Intercostals
- ▼ Internal Intercostals

Expiration (forced)
- ▼ Transverse Abdominis
- ▼ Rectus Abdominis
- ★ External Intercostals
- ★ Internal Intercostals
- ★ Quadratus Lumborum
- ▼ External Obliques
- ▼ Internal Obliques
- ★ Muscles of the neck and shoulder

Major muscles of the body

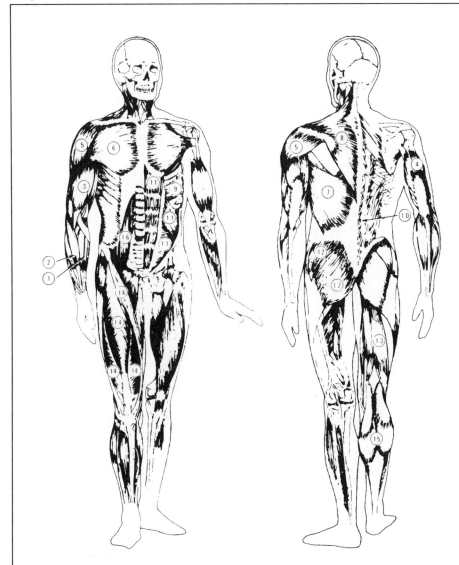

1. Forearm flexors
2. Brachioradialis
3. Biceps
4. Triceps
5. Deltoid
6. Pectoral muscles
7. Latissimus Dorsi
8. Trapezius
9. Serratus anterior
10. Erector spinae
    (spinal extensors)
11. Abdominal muscles
    a. Internal and external
       obliques
    b. Rectus abdominis
    c. Transversalis
12. Gluteal muscles
13. Hamstrings
14. Quadriceps muscles
15. Gastrocnemius, soleus
    muscles
16. Iliopsoas (under abdominal muscles)

Study Questions / Learning Activities

1. Differentiate between the three anatomical planes of movement.

2. Perform an anatomical movement and have a partner identify the name of the movement in anatomical terms (anatomical charades).

3. Identify what anatomical movements and muscle groups are used in wheel-chair propulsion.

4. List and define seven types of roles that muscle may respond in.

5. Differentiate between the three different types of muscle contractions.

6. On a schematic of muscles of the human body, identify the major muscle groups.

7. Identify the various body positions used for performing exercises.

References

Hay, J. G., & Reid, J. G. (1982). *The anatomical and mechanical bases of human motion.* Englewood Cliffs, NJ: Prentice-Hall.

Hoppenfeld, S. (1976). *Physical examination of the spine and extremities.* New York: Appleton-Century-Crofts.

Logan, G. A., & McKinney, W. C. (1982). *Anatomic kinesiology.* Dubuque: Wm. C. Brown.

Smith, J. C. (1974). *Laboratory manual for human neuromuscular anatomy.* University of California, Los Angeles.

CHAPTER 3

Contraindicated Exercises

The purpose of this chapter is to present the reasons why certain popular exercises and techniques are now considered contraindicated for many adults. Where appropriate, alternative exercises or techniques have been suggested. An important point to remember is that any exercise can become contraindicated if improperly performed or prescribed for the wrong reason. Exercises should always be performed utilizing neutral spine technique. Three questions to ask when selecting exercises for an individual are:

1. What is the purpose of the exercise?
2. Is the exercise necessary for achieving this participant's program goals?
3. Can the exercise be performed safely by this participant without violating principles of good biomechanics? If not, what is an alternative exercise?

Circumduction/Hyperextension of the Cervical Spine ("head circles")

Rational: Strains the supporting ligaments which maintain stability in the cervical spine. Causes compression of the intervertebral disk and impingement of the spinous processes. When combined with the degenerative changes that occur with aging (e.g., loss of synovial fluid, osteoporosis), the individual is more susceptible to neck injury.

Alternative: Perform isometric exercises for cervical flexion and rotation right and left to strengthen the muscles about the cervical spine.

Head Circles

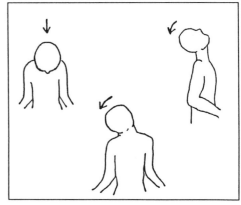

Trunk Circling

Rational: Hyperextension of the lumbar spine reinforces lordosis, especially for those with weak abdominals. Flexing the spine from a standing position with straight legs dramatically increases the intervertebral disc pressure in the lumbar area. Both directions of movement compress the intervertebral disc which has already thinned with age, creating a greater susceptibility to herniation of the nucleus pulposus. Lateral flexion usually results in an inadvertent rounding of the upper back and a relaxed abdomen.

Trunk Circling

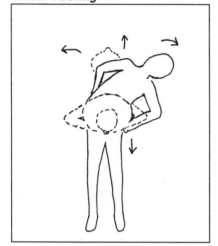

Alternative: Omit flexion and hyperextension. During lateral flexion, use a diagonal reach with the heel, buttocks, low back, upper back, and head pressed against a wall (Stevenson, 1983). This maneuver requires a pelvic tilt or contraction of the abdomen. Performing the stretch in a sitting position further eliminates any uncontrolled hyperextension of the lumbar spine (include a pelvic tilt).

Shoulder Stand

Rational: Strains the muscles and ligaments of the cervical and thoracic spine and reinforces the postures of foward head and kyphosis.

Alternative: Exercises which stretch the hamstrings and low back from a long sitting or supine-lying position.

Shoulder Stand

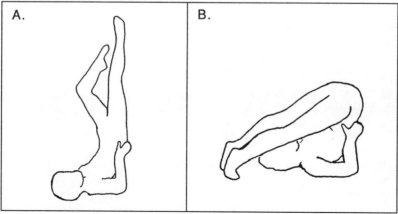

A.

B.

Prone Hyperextension of the Spine ("prone trunk raise")

Rational: Compresses the lumbar intervertebral discs, stretches the abdominal muscles, and encourages the posture of lordosis. The purpose of this exercise is to strengthen the low back muscles; yet, weakness in this area is seldom encountered in the general population, with the exception of paralytic conditions and flat back posture.

Alternative: To strengthen the hip extensors, assume a four-point position, resting on the elbows instead of the hands. Extend one leg and lift it up and down, keeping the abdominals contracted and being careful not to hyperextend the spine or hip. If the extensor muscles of the spine require strengthening (e.g., polio, trunk paresis), the individual should assume the prone-lying position with arms extended out to the sides with palms down. The shoulders and arms should be raised slightly off the mat, pinching the shoulder blades together and rotating the thumbs up toward the ceiling (shoulder is externally rotating).

Prone Trunk Raise

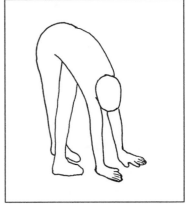

If the individual has strength in the hip extensors, a hook-lying position can be assumed. The individual then lifts the hips off the mat, contracting the extensor muscles of the spine and hip.

Standing Toe Touches with Straight Legs

Toe Touches

Rational: Hyperextends the posterior joint capsule and ligaments of the knee. Increases intervertebral disc pressure in lumbar region during spinal flexion. Bouncing from this position may trigger stretch reflexes, resulting in muscular strain. In addition, rounding of the upper back is encouraged from this posture.

Alternative: Hamstring stretches from a long sitting or supine position.

Bilateral Straight Leg Raises

Rational: The anatomical movement involved in this exercise is hip flexion. The prime mover for hip flexion is the iliopsoas muscle group (iliacus and psoas combined) which originates from the vertebrae in the low back (twelfth thoracic and all lumbar) and inserts onto the lesser trochanter of the femur. During the leg raise, the spine hyperextends from the great pull of the iliopsoas, especially when the abdominals are weak and can not counteract the anterior tilt of the pelvis. Extreme muscular soreness and strain may result. It should be remembered that the abdominals only serve to stabilize the trunk and pelvis during hip flexion from supine - they are not the prime movers in this exercise.

Leg Raises

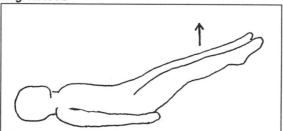

Alternative: Abdominal curls from a supine-hook position. The trunk should be raised only high enough for the scapula to clear the floor.

Sit-Up with Feet Held and Hands Behind Head

Rational: Holding the feet during sit-ups increases the activation of the hip flexors to pull the trunk up, rather than the abdominal muscles. This technique encourages a hyper-extended posture of the low back (lordosis) and may cause muscular soreness and strain. Holding the hands behind the head may contribute to forward head and kyphosis, as well as cause pressure on the nerve roots in the cervical area. In addition, do not use an incline plane. This also places a strain on the low back, due to the extra work required of the hip flexors.

Alternative: Abdominal curls from a supine-hook position without the feet held. Hands should be placed across the chest or at sides of the head with the elbows out. Do not interlock the fingers at the back of the head.

Sit-ups with Straight Legs

Rational: This exercise primarily involves the hip flexors; thus, the same mechanical stresses result that are described in exercise #6.

Alternative: See strength exercises for abdominals in Chapter 6.

Ballistic Stretching

Rational: Rapid "bounce" stretching of muscles will activate the muscle spindles, thus eliciting the stretch reflex. This reaction causes the stretched muscle to contract and may induce strain or micro-tears of muscle fibers.

Alternative: See Chapter 7 for correct stretching techniques and specific exercises.

Trunk Twists from a Standing Position

Rational: Strains the lumbar region and possibly the knee. Torque generated by the trunk must be absorbed in the knee. Never allow an individual to flex forward and then twist the trunk as nerve impingement may result.

Alternative: Perform the trunk twist very slowly in a sitting position. The knee can better absorb torque when flexed because of its greater capacity for rotation in a sitting position.

Isometric Exercises

Rational: Contraindicated for individuals over 40 years of age or those with a history of cardiovascular pathology, particularly high blood pressure. These exercises have a tendency to raise the systolic blood pressure to unsafe levels, especially isometric arm exercise, due to increased peripheral resistance to blood flow.

Full Flexion of the Knee Joint from a Standing Position (deep knee bends or "squats")

Rational: Creates an excessive stretch on the collateral and cruciate ligaments of the knee joint and may pinch the joint cartilage. Repetitive lengthening of the ligaments may lead to instability of the knee joint.

Alternative: Squat no more than half the distance to full flexion (i.e., thighs are parallel to the floor).

Bench Press Performed with the Feet on the Floor

Rational: Creates hyperextension of the lumbar spine which reinforces lordosis. During the maneuver, intervertebral disc pressure increases dramatically, predisposing one to low back injury.

Alternative: Place the feet on the bench from a hook-lying position or against a wall so that the hips and knees are flexed to 90 degrees. This flattens the lumbar spine by removing the pull of the iliopsoas upon the vertebra.

Bench Press

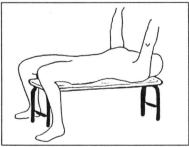

Alternative

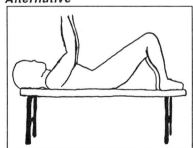

Hip Flexor Stretches

Rational: These particular stretches compress the intervertebral lumbar discs and reinforce the posture of lordosis. Hyperextension of the cervical discs may occur.

Alternative: While standing and holding onto a chair with the left hand, grasp the right ankle with the right hand from behind, flexing at the knee.

Hip Flexion

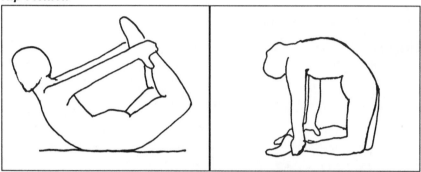

Hurdle Stretch

Hurdle Stretch
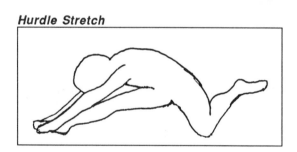

Rational: Strains the medial collateral ligament of the internally rotated and flexed knee, especially when the iliotibial band is adaptively shortened.

Alternative: Externally rotate the flexed knee to remove the strain.

Holding the Breath During Exercise

Rational: Decreases venous return of blood to the heart, possibly resulting in dizziness or fainting.

Alternative: Breath rythmically; exhale with the lift or effort; inhale with the lowering of weight. Breathe naturally and do not force the exhale.

Wearing Rubberized Suits During Workout

Rational: Prevents the normal physiologic mechanisms of body cooling from occurring (i.e., evaporation, conduction). May lead to a rise in core body temperature.

Immediate Rest After Intense Exercise

Rational: Prevents adequate venous return of blood. Blood lactate is not recycled.

Alternative: Continue with low aerobic exercise (e.g., walking) to encourage venous return and recycling of blood lactate.

Military Press

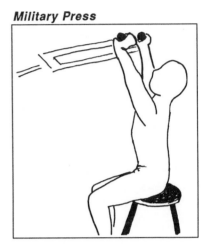

Military Press

Rational: Individual often hyperextends spine during the lift, causing excessive compression of the intervertebral lumbar discs. This posture is more likely to occur when the anterior region of the shoulder is limited in flexibility.

Alternative: Pointing the chin down during the lift will help reduce excessive lumbar curve. Perform Upright Rows from a standing position. See Chapter 6 for a description of this exercise.

Prone Flies from a Standing Position (shoulder horizontal abduction)

Rational: Compression forces to the L-4 and L-5 intervertebral discs increase approximately 3 1/2 times when an individual assumes this straight leg position (without weights!). Exercises with or without weights should never be performed from this "7" position.

Alternative: Assume a prone position on a low bench. Long extensor muscles of the back will be relaxed and will not assist in lifting from this position.

Prone Flies

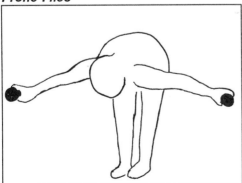

Alternative

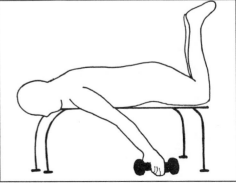

Study Questions / Learning Activities

1. What three questions should be asked when selecting exercises for an individual?

2. Why should the knees and hips be flexed for any exercise performed in the supine position?

3. After reading this chapter, which region of the body appears most vulnerable to improper exercises? Why?

4. Describe any exercises you have performed in the past that would now be considered contraindicated and state the reasons why.

References

Algra, B. (1982). An in-depth analysis of the bench press. *National Strength and Conditioning Association Journal*, October-November.

Allsop, K.G. (1977). Potential hazards of abdominal exercises. *Journal of Health, Physical Education, Recreation, and Dance, 45*, 89-91.

Alter, J. (1983). *Surviving exercises*. Boston: Houghton Mifflin.

Flint, M. M. (1965). An electromyographic comparison of the function of the iliacus and the rectus abdominis muscles. *Physical Therapy, 45*, 248-253.

Flint, M. M., & Gudgell, J. (1965). Electromyographic study of abdominal muscular activity during exercise. *Research Quarterly, 36*, 29-37.

Flint, M. M. (1965). Abdominal muscle involvement during the performance of various forms of sit-up exercise. *American Journal of Physical Medicine, 44*, 224-234.

Kendall, F. P. (1965). A criticism of current tests and exercises for physical fitness. *Physical Therapy, 45*, 187-197.

Kendall, H. O. (1968). Developing and maintaining good posture. *Journal of Physical Therapy, 48*(4).

Rasch, P. J., & Burke, R. K. (1971, 4th ed.). *Kinesiology and applied anatomy*. Philadelphia: W. B. Saunders.

Stevenson, E. (1973). *Physique magic*. Sacramento: California State University, Sacramento.

Stevenson, E. (1981). Recycled exercise. *California Association for Health, Physical Education, Recreation, and Dance (CAHPERD) Journal Times, 44*(2).

Stevenson, E. (1983). The shoulder stand. *California Association for Health, Physical Education, Recreation, and Dance (CAHPERD) Journal Times, 45*(6), 19-20.

Stevenson, E. (1983). The shoulder stand. *Journal of the California Association for Health, Physical Education, Recreation, and Dance, 45*(6), 19-20.

Stevenson, E. (1987). The shoulder stand. *California Association for Health, Physical Education, Recreation, and Dance (CAHPERD) Journal Times, 49*(8), 16-17.

4

Transfers, Orthotics, and Ambulation Aids

Transfers

Transfer refers to the relocation of an individual from one surface to another and can be classified as either "standing" or "sitting." Variations on these two types of transfers depend on the capabilities of the individual and the type of surface he/she is transferring to. Many persons have developed their own individual technique for executing a transfer and this preference should be discussed before the assistant or instructor attempts to help.

General Guidelines for Performing Transfers

1. Reduce the distance between the transfer surfaces. Removing arm rests and detachable footrests will permit closer positioning of the person to the transfer surface.
2. Always secure wheelchair brakes. They are essential for safety and stability.
3. Transfer to a surface of equal height if possible. A sliding board may be used to eliminate the gap between the two surfaces. Be sure to stabilize the sliding board on both transfer surfaces.
4. When transferring an individual with one-sided involvement (e.g., hemiplegia), position the wheelchair alongside the table on the individual's stronger side. Provide assistance from the weaker side.
5. Keep a wide base of support. Placing one foot ahead of the other allows you to shift your weight more easily.
6. Keep your back straight while flexing at the hips and knees during the transfer. Hold the person as close as possible and lift with the thigh muscles, extending at the knees and hips, not the back.
7. If possible, allow the individual to view the surface to which he/she is being transferred to.
8. To increase the stability of the wheelchair, place the casters in a forward position.

Performance Requirements

For Standing Transfers

The individual should possess partial or full weight-bearing capabilities when attempting a "stand and pivot" transfer. Although it is possible to perform this type of transfer with an individual possessing complete lower extremity paralysis, it is generally not recommended in an APE program for safety and liability reasons. To maximize the safety of participants, it is suggested that a sitting transfer be used instead. If a participant is overweight or evidences a great deal of spasticity, a sitting transfer should also be considered.

For Sitting Transfers

1. **One-man** (front-facing). The individual should possess sufficient muscular strength to depress the shoulder and extend the elbow (C-7 nerve root level), lifting his/her body weight off of a surface.
2. **Two-man** (one man front-facing and one man back-facing). This transfer is used when the participant is overweight, excessively spastic, or lacks both weight-bearing and upper extremity strength (e.g., quadriplegia from spinal cord injury).

Description of Specific Transfers

Pull to Stand in Parallel Bars

1. The participant should position the buttocks close to the edge of the wheelchair seat. Place your hands either underneath the buttocks or around the waist. Participant places hands on parallel bars with elbows extended.
2. As the participant leans the trunk forward and pulls with the arms, shift your weight backward and pull the participant to a stand.
3. Be sure to keep participant's knees blocked until standing is stabilized.

Pull to Stand in Parallel Bars

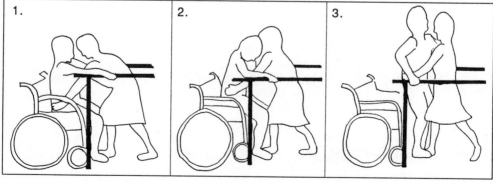

Stand and Pivot

1. Slide the participant forward until the buttocks are close to the edge of the wheelchair seat. Feet should be planted on the floor. Place your hands underneath the participant's buttocks. If the participant is strong enough, his/her arms should be placed around your shoulders. If not, the participant's arms should hang in front of the body. Block the participant's feet so they do not slide out from underneath. Also squeeze or block the knees to prevent them from buckling during the transfer. Have the participant hook his/her chin over your shoulder. Allow the participant to view the surface he/she is being transferred to.
2. Rock the participant's trunk forward and lift him/her high enough to clear the wheelchair. Pivot the participant, preventing sliding of feet or buckling of knees.
3. As the participant is lowered to the mat, slide one hand up from the buttocks to the mid-back to stabilize in the sitting position.

Stand and Pivot

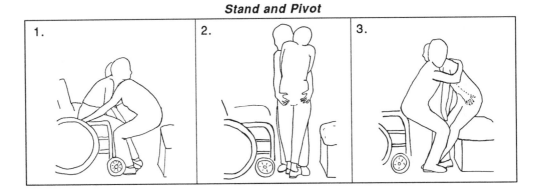

Sitting Transfer (one man, front-facing)

1. Place the chair approximately 45 degrees to the treatment table. Place the participant's legs (extended) on the table.
2. Places your hands around the participant's waist or underneath the buttocks. Lift as the participant extends his/her elbows.
3. Swing the participant over to the mat, using the feet as the pivot point.

Sitting Transfer (one-man, front-facing)

1.   2.   3.

Sitting Transfer (two-man)

1. Position the wheelchair at a 45 degree angle to the treatment table. Have the participant flex his/her elbows and place the forearms against the chest. Standing behind the participant, bring your arms underneath the armpits and grasp the forearms. Alternative hand grip: grasp the left forearm with your right hand and vice versa. The second assistant places both hands underneath the legs in a cradle-like fashion. An alternative transfer may be indicated for a person with subluxating shoulder joints.
2. On the count of three, both assistants lift the participant to the mat. The back-facing assistant should lift by pressing the arms into the chest, rather than pulling up into the armpits. Slowly position the participant on the mat to prevent spasticity from occurring.

Sitting Transfer (two-man)

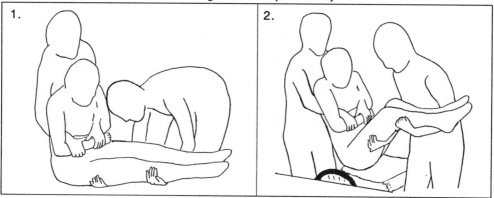

Lower Extremity Orthotics

Primarily three types of lower extremity braces or orthoses have been designed for assisting in standing and ambulation: short leg braces, long leg braces, and hip braces. The purposes of these orthotics are three-fold (Venn, Morganstern, & Dykes, 1979):

1. To support body weight (e.g., muscular dystrophy).
2. To control involuntary movement (e.g., cerebral palsy).
3. To correct or prevent deformities (e.g., Legg-Perthes disease).

Checklists evaluating the condition of orthotics, prosthetics, and wheelchairs may be obtained from an article by Venn, Morganstern, and Dykes (1979).

Types

Short Leg Brace

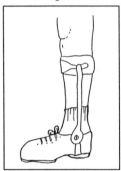

Ankle-Foot Orthosis (AFO) or Short Leg Brace

- Used for conditions which occur at the ankle joint (e.g., drop-foot).
- Controls plantarflexion, dorsiflexion, inversion, and eversion. Prevents medial/lateral instability.
- Consists of a metal or plastic upright bar attached to a shoe with a cuff around the calf of the leg.

Long Leg Brace

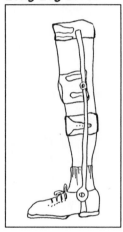

Knee-Ankle-Foot Orthosis (KAFO) or Long Leg Brace

- Prevents hyperextension and flexion of the knee resulting from weak quadriceps or hamstrings.
- Consists of an extension of the AFO with a cuff around the upper thigh. A sliding metal lock is attached at the knee joint (locked when standing/ ambulating and unlocked when sitting).

Long Leg Brace with Pelvic Band

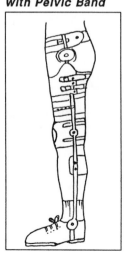

Hip-Knee-Ankle-Foot Orthosis (HKAFO) or Long Leg Brace with Pelvic Band

- Consists of an extension of the KAFO with a pelvic band attached.
- Controls the six movements of the hip (i.e., flexion, extension, abduction, adduction, internal rotation, and external rotation). Can be unlocked to allow for flexion and extension.

Ambulation Aids

People with a lower extremity disability usually require some form of assistive device during ambulation. Canes, crutches, and walkers serve as extensions which permit the upper extremities to transmit force to the floor, providing support for the lower extremities and improving balance. Because of the diversity of ambulation aids, their prescription and fit should be carefully evaluated by a physician or licensed physical therapist. The person with a disability should receive instruction in their use, including proper gait pattern, ascending and descending stairs, and sitting and arising. Pre-ambulation exercises and training are often necessary for persons with severe disabilities (Jebsen, 1967).

Typical walker

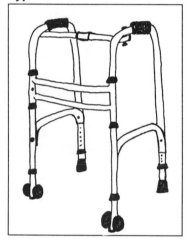

Walkers

Walkers are indicated when an individual lacks balance, strength and/or coordination (e.g., stroke, cerebral palsy). Some models can be folded up for storage or travel. During ambulation, the individual lifts the walker up and places it in front of him/her, and then walks forward between the bars. There are several different types of walkers, including some models with rollers and/or adjustable seats.

Types of Walkers

1. **Walkerette**. This model has runners attached to the bars and is pushed forward along the floor. It is not lifted by the user like a standard walker.
2. **Roller Walker**. This model has wheels on the front legs so that the individual can raise the rear legs off the floor and roll the walker forward.
3. **Crutch Walker**. This model has crutches attached to the horizontal bars to support body weight. It also has a seat for the individual to rest on when fatigued. The crutches can be removed or draped to the sides when not in use.

Crutches

The use of crutches requires more balance, strength and coordination than a walker. One or two crutches may be used, depending upon the extent of support needed. Chapter 9 details the different types of gait patterns that can be employed with crutches and canes.

Types of Crutches

1. **Axillary crutch.**
2. **Canadian, Lofstrand or Elbow Extension Crutch.** This crutch has no shoulder rest and is usually prescribed for persons who can ambulate using the four-point crutch gait and need support for weak arm musculature.
3. **Gutter Crutch.** This crutch has been designed for persons with a significant flexion deformity at the elbow, painful wrist, or very poor hand function. The forearm may be secured to the crutch by a velcro strap or other fastening.

Axillary Crutch   *Canadian Crutch*   *Gutter Crutch*

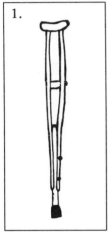
1.

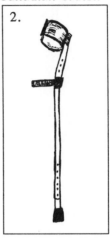
2.

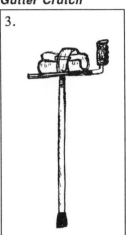
3.

Crutch Adjustment

The crutch height should always be adjustable. It is also preferable to use crutches that are adjustable with respect to length and position of the arm support (Cash, 1976). The length of the axillary crutch should extend from a point two inches below the axilla to a point near the foot indicated in the illustration. The height of the hand grip should be positioned so that the elbow is flexed between 15-30 degrees. The wrists should be hyperextended and the weight borne on the palms. When fitting axillary crutches, it is essential that the user be instructed **not** to bear weight on the axillary bar. This may cause compression of the radial nerve, resulting in paralysis which may take months to resolve. The true purpose of this bar is to provide lateral stability of the crutch via pressure against the chest wall (Jebsen, 1967). Regularly check crutch tips for worn areas, cracking, or plugging of the grooves with lint and dirt.

Crutch Adjustment

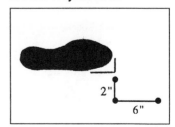

2"

6"

Canes

Canes are generally prescribed when some weight bearing can be taken on the affected extremity or when only mild balance deficits exist. It is difficult for a person to develop a normal walking pattern with one cane. Because a cane supports approximately 20-25% of the body weight, the tendency is to lean the body over the cane and shorten the stride on that side.

Types of Canes

1. **Standard Cane**. This model is made of wood or aluminum with a C-curved handle. A telescoping cane is available which can be adjusted to between 22-38".
2. **Tripod Cane**. This model has three prongs at the end of the shaft with flexible rubber sockets, allowing for movement of the shaft while the prongs remain in contact with the ground during ambulation.
3. **Quad Cane**. This model has four prongs that come in contact with the floor. It is adjustable in length and provides maximum support and balance with four contact points on the ground. This device is frequently prescribed for those with athetoid cerebral palsy.

Cane Adjustment

The length of the cane is determined by measuring the vertical distance from the greater trochanter to the floor. The elbow should be flexed approximately 15-30 degrees. The cane should be held in the hand opposite the affected leg. During ambulation the cane should be held fairly close to the side to avoid leaning.

Wheelchairs

The market currently offers a wide selection of wheelchairs, from heavy duty chairs to light sport models with racing tires. In addition, a variety of sizes are available such as Adult, Narrow-Adult, Tall, Junior, and Children's sizes. Some companies will even customize the size of a chair to the individual. *Sport and Spokes*, a magazine for athletes with disabilities, publishes an annual review of the latest models of sport wheelchairs. A physician or physical therapist familiar with the sizes, models, and components of wheelchairs will prescribe a suitable chair for an individual.

Assistants should become familiar with the basic components of the wheelchair and their operation. The following is a description of the most basic components of a typical wheelchair. There are many additional accessories which can be attached to the wheelchair to enhance its effectiveness to the user.

1. **Wheels**. For ease of ride over outdoor terrain (soft, sandy or rough ground), pneumatic tires are recommended.
2. **Handrims**. Handrims are connected to the wheels to allow the user to move his wheelchair without injuring the hands. They come in a variety of sizes

and types, depending on the sport and ability of the individual. Rubber-coated handrims are available to persons with quadriplegia. For the person with severe limitations of grip, a handrim consisting of eight rubber-tipped vertical projections is available.

3. **Backrest.** The height of the backrest depends on the height of the user and the degree of trunk stability. Reclining backrests are available for those who need to be in a partially or fully reclined position.

4. **Armrests.** Armrests may be either detached or fixed. Detachable armrests easily lift off to allow the convenience of side transfers. The height of the armrests can usually be adjusted to accommodate the changes created by a wheelchair cushion.

5. **Wheel-locks (brakes).** These brakes prevent the wheelchair from rolling forward or backward on inclines.

6. **Casters.** These small wheels sit towards the front of the wheelchair. Casters are most stable when they have anti-flutter caster bearings. Casters also come in the following styles: heavy-duty, light-weight, and pneumatic (for a cushioned ride with a freer roll).

7. **Front Rigging.** This consists of a footrest or legrest. The latter is used with those who need the legs elevated. Both types of rigging typically have a swing-away feature which allows for a close approach to transfer surfaces. Heel-loops help prevent feet from sliding off of the footplate.

Study Questions / Learning Activities

1. List eight general guidelines for performing transfers.

2. Describe the abilities needed to perform a standing and sitting transfers.

3. With partners, demonstrate a (1) transfer from a wheelchair to standing in parallel bars, and (2) two-man sitting transfer.

4. Identify the three general purposes of lower extremity orthotics.

5. Identify the specific purposes of AFO, KAFO, and HKAFO braces.

6. List and describe the basic components of the wheelchar.

7. Obtain a vendor catalog of ambulatory aids and determine what abilities each device was intended for.

8. Visit a local wheelchair sporting event (e.g., road race, track meet, basketball game, tennis). Note or photograph all the different types of wheelchairs and accessories you find.

References

Bromley, I. (1981). *Tetraplegia and paraplegia. A guide for physiotherapists.* New York: Churchill Livingstone.

Cash, J. E. (1976). *A textbook of medical conditions for physiotherapists.* Philadelphia: J. B. Lippincott.

Jebsen, R. (1967). Use and abuse of ambulation aids. *Journal of the American Medical Association, 199(1),* 63-65.

Sorenson, L. & Ulrich, P.G. (1977). *Ambulation Guides for Nurses, Revised Edition.* Minneapolis: Sister Kenny Institute.

Venn, J., Morganstern, L., & Dykes, M. K. (1979). Checklists for evaluating the fit and function of orthoses, prostheses, and wheelchairs in the classroom. *Teaching Exceptional Children, 11*(2), 51-56.

5

Effective Teaching

Optimal learning occurs when the teaching style is congruent with the characteristics of the learner. No single teaching style, strategy, approach, or method is a panacea for all instructional situations. Effective teachers appropriately adapt teaching styles to match various learning styles of their students. In post-secondary APE programs, instructors and assistants are faced with the challenge of facilitating learning for a group of individuals who possess various disabling conditions and learning styles. Understanding the learning process in these situations is crucial and means the difference between mediocre and effective programs. This chapter will review the different learning styles one may encounter in APE programs and present instructional strategies for facilitating optimal learning.

General Principles of Learning

There are numerous principles which affect the participant's rate and amount of learning. The teacher of adults must understand these principles if he/she wishes to be successful and effective.

Law of Effect

People tend to accept and repeat those responses which are pleasant and satisfying and avoid those which are not.

Nothing Succeeds Like Success

Make every effort to see that participants achieve some success during each class.

Law of Primacy

First impressions are lasting. Make those initial class meetings meaningful.

Law of Practice

The more often an act is repeated, the quicker the skill is established.

Law of Disuse

A skill not practiced or knowledge not used with be forgotten quickly. Important skills and concepts need to be reviewed.

Law of Vigor

A dramatic or exciting learning experience is more likely to be remembered than a routine or boring experience. Let your teaching come alive. Use vivid examples and participate with the participants. Remember that humor is a useful teaching tool.

Accommodating Learning Style Preferences

Each individual, whether disabled or not, has a preferential learning style involving a dominant sensory channel. To foster the learning experience, the instructor needs to know the learning style of each participant. Table 5-1 will provide clues to decide if a participant is primarily a visual, auditory, or kinesthetic learner. A participant will learn quicker if he/she is taught through his/her dominant sensory mode.

Table 5-1.   *Accommodating Learning Style Preferences*

Primary Learning Styles	Instructional and Learning Implications
Visual Preference	Provide an unobstructed vision to teacher and the board or demonstrations. Visual learners learn best when the instructor: • Creates an image through descriptive language. • Uses examples and analogies. • Supplements lectures with: Filmstrips/, Movies/Slides/Videos, Pictures, Graphs, Observation of Others • Distribute structured outlines prior to the lecture. • Distribute script prior to movie/slide show. • Provide written directions.
Auditory Preference	The auditory learner learns best by: • Lectures. • Simple and consistent language. • Oral directions. • Discussions and panels. • Question/answer sessions. Comprehends reading material by reading out loud or by talking to self.
Kinesthetic Preference	The kinesthethic learner learns best by: • Role playing and simulation exercises. • Experiments/demonstrations. • Movement experiences and use of body parts. • Use of tactile models: raised line drawings, clay models, etc.

Instructional Strategies

The importance of assistant/participant interactions cannot be over-emphasized. The primary function of the assistant is to hasten the participant's cognitive, psychomotor, and affective development as they relate to physical education. Assistants should be aware of the types of interactions which foster the participant's learning, motivation to exercise, and attendance. The following section describes instructional strategies in the visual, auditory, and kinesthetic/tactile domains (adapted from McKenzie, 1984). If a participant has a weak sensory channel - visual, auditory, or kinesthetic/tactile - then a multisensory approach is warranted. This approach makes use of all of the senses to promote and reinforce the learning of knowledge or skills.

Visual Domain

1. Demonstrate a skill whenever possible.
2. Tell the participants what to look for in your demonstrations.
3. Be sure everyone in the group can see you.
4. Maintain eye contact when speaking to participants.
5. Use diagrams if necessary.
6. Use visual cues to enhance body awareness and coordinated movement (e.g., footprints placed on the floor; stickers placed on the body or equipment; pointing to a body part; arrows or lines on the floor).

Auditory Domain

1. Whenever possible, provide the participant with facts or background information regarding exercises or procedures.
2. If needed, verbally direct a participant to perform a task.
3. Allow participants with hearing impairments to see your mouth and hand gestures. Do not over-exaggerate mouth movements.
4. Provide corrective skill feedback - information regarding how to correct an inadequate performance. Knowledge of results leads to increased learning.
5. Provide positive skill feedback - tell participants what they did correctly to reinforce the likelihood the skill being correctly performed again.
6. Ask questions regarding discomfort during exercises (e.g., pain during passive range of motion; pain during cardiovascular training). This information alerts the assistant to signs of exercise distress and provides feedback regarding his/her technique. The assistant should also ask questions regarding exercises or procedures for the purpose of testing the participant's knowledge.
7. Listen to the participant's questions, responses, or attempts at conversation.
8. Utilize praise, vocal intonation, claps, gestures, and expressions to activate or intensify motor performances or foster appropriate behavior.
9. Use simple verbal cues to assist the participant in better visualizing the movement.

Kinesthetic/Tactile Domain

1. Manually guide a participant with a visual impairment or apraxia through the desired motions.
2. Physically assist a participant whenever needed (e.g., manual assistance which enables a participant to reach full range of motion).
3. Tap the body part to facilitate movement in the correct direction.

Characteristic Behaviors of Effective Teachers

Effective teachers. . . .

1. Hold and project high expectations for participant success.
2. Maximize opportunities for participants to engage in learning experiences.
3. Manage their own time and organize the classroom efficiently.
4. Pace the curriculum to maximize participant success.
5. Engage in active teaching with all participants whether individually or in groups of varying size.
6. Work toward mastery of knowledge and skills by systematically monitoring participant progress and providing feedback.
7. Are sensitive to differences in rate of learning and type of teacher-participant contact required.
8. Provide a supportive learning environment that is characterized by warmth and personal support.
9. Select equipment and activities that are appropriate for the developmental level of the participant.
10. Remember that a participant's self-esteem is more important than any exercise or activity.
11. Think of what the participants **can do**, not what they **cannot do**.
12. Are well prepared — know the material, know the participants, and know the appropriate teaching style.

Professional Conduct of Assistants

1. Attend the program regularly. The assistants are generally responsible for one or two participants. If the assistant is absent, participants may have difficulty completing their exercise programs. Therefore, dependable attendance by the assistant is critical. The instructor should be informed in advance of an absence.
2. Be punctual.
3. Use appropriate language and terminology (see Chapter 1).
4. Refrain from unnecessary chatting with fellow assistants.
5. Wear appropriate clothing.

6. Maintain proper posture.
7. Respect the participant's privacy. The assistant will often have access to information about the particpant's disability, age, and medications. This information should not be shared with friends.
8. Do not let a particpant's mood determine your mood.
9. Demonstrate a sense of enjoyment. This practice facilitates the participant's enjoyment of the exercise session.
10. Be creative. Try to modify the exercise program (**with approval from the instructor**) until it is really individualized for the participant.
11. Measure and record performance. The assistant should constantly be engaged in observing a participant's performance and recording the data on the exercise program card.

Study Questions / Learning Activities

1. Are you predominantly a visual, auditory, or kinesthetic learner? On what do you base your answer? Give some specific examples of how you learn best.

2. Ask your family members the same question in #1. Does a preferential learning style run in your family?

3. Describe your first teaching experience. What aspects of the lesson could have been improved?

4. Identify someone you think is an effective teacher and list characteristics that contribute to his/her effectiveness.

5. Select several strength and flexibility exercises. Practice teaching a partner these exercises, using a multisensory approach.

References

Fait, H., & Dunn, J. (1989, 6th ed.). *Special physical education - adapted, individualized and developmental.* Dubuque: Wm. C. Brown.

McKenzie, T. (1984). Lecture notes from Analysis of Teaching Behavior. San Diego State University.

6

Assessment and Programming for Muscular Strength and Endurance

Why Assess?

Assessment is one of the more important aspects of an exercise program; yet, it is often the most neglected due to lack of evaluation tools, expertise, and time. Physical and motor assessment of a participant with disabilities is vital to an adapted physical education program for the following reasons:

1. It establishes the participant's current level or performance (i.e., functional ability).
2. It allows the instructor to plan individualized goals and prescribe feasible, safe, and beneficial exercises.
3. Upon post-testing, it enables the participant to see either the progress that has been made or maintenance that has been kept. Ocassionally, regression will be noted in the case of degenerative conditions.

Some assessment tools are not suitable for all disabilities. For example, the Manual Muscle Test is suitable for testing participants with lower motoneuron lesions such as polio, but is inappropriate for any participant with an upper motoneuron lesion. In addition, the participant's posture and starting position for selected activities should be considered in the assessment. It is also important to note any compensatory mechanisms or muscle substitutions that occur during a movement.

NOTE

Before conducting any form of evaluation, please refer to Chapter 15 for Contra-indications to Exercise Testing and Reasons for Terminating an Exercise Test.

Assessment of Muscular Strength and Endurance

Developing and maintaining adequate levels of muscular strength and endurance are essential in facilitating independent living skills, preventing disuse syndrome, and avoiding acute or chronic injury (e.g., low back pain). Prior to beginning a strength training regime, some form of evaluation is necessary to determine which techniques and adaptations will be used, as well as the initial amount of sets, repetitions, and load to be lifted for exercise.

Definitions

Strength: The maximal amount of force that can be elicited in a single or several voluntary contractions (Sharkey, 1979).

Endurance: The ability to exert submaximal contractions repeatedly (Sharkey, 1979).

Muscular strength and endurance fall along the same continuum and are usually distinguished by the number of repetitions involved (see illustration below).

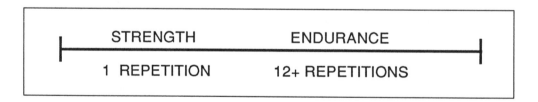

Methods and devices currently used to assess muscular strength and endurance in adults with disabilities include manual muscle testing, grip strength dynamometers and cynamometers (isometric), repetition maximum with weights (isotonic), static cable tensiometry (isometric), and isokinetic dynamometers (Davis et al., 1981). Most of these methods are discussed below. Many other tests exist for assessing muscular strength and endurance. The reader is referred to books by Haskins (1972), Fait and Dunn (1984), and Sherrill (1986) for additional fitness tests. Unfortunately, few norms exist for adults, especially those with disabilities.

Manual Muscle Testing

Manual muscle testing is used by therapists, athletic trainers, and adapted physical educators to assess strength of isolated muscle (e.g., tibialis anterior) or groups of muscles (e.g., dorsiflexors). It is a valuable method because it requires no equipment other than a plinth and may be the only method for testing when paresis, contractures, or incoordination are present. However, it is a method which requires an advanced knowledge of muscles and their actions, as well as practical expertise in positioning and technique. Therefore, it should not be attempted without rigorous training prior to its utilization. The test is inappropriate for participants with upper motoneuron lesions evidencing spasticity. The technique is executed by having the evaluator apply resistance while the participant performs an anatomical movement. Muscular strength is rated by the evaluator according to the standard muscle grading chart in Table 6-1 (Hoppenfeld, 1976). For specific details regarding the positions and procedures used in manual muscle testing, refer to the text by Daniels and Worthingham (1972) listed in the reference section at the end of this chapter.

Table 6-1. *Muscle Grading Chart*

Gradations	Criteria
5 - Normal	Complete range of motion against gravity with full resistance.
4 - Good	Complete range of motion against gravity with some resistance.
3 - Fair	Complete range of motion against gravity.
2 - Poor	Complete range of motion with gravity eliminated.
1 - Trace	Evidence of slight contractility. No joint motion.
0 - Zero	No evidence of contractility.

Another quick version of the manual muscle test is the "break test". This technique involves placing each muscle group in its maximally shortened position and determining how much resistance is needed to "break" the participant out of the position. The shortened position is used because (1) it is generally the weakest portion of the range of motion and (2) it demonstrates if the participant can move through the range of motion against gravity. Specific positions and procedures used during this test may be found in Hoppenfeld (1976) listed in the reference section at the end of this chapter.

General Guidelines for the Break Test

1. If possible, each muscle group should be initially tested in an anti-gravity position.
2. The muscle group should be placed at the end-range (i.e., maximally shortened) position for the break test, with the exception of elbow extensors, shoulder flexors and abductors, and forearm supinators and pronators. Use the mid-range position for these muscle groups.
3. One hand of the evaluator should stabilize the joint to be tested. The remaining hand will act as the resistor.

4. The evaluator should gradually build up to the maximal resistance that the participant can overcome.
5. Do not perform this test on a spastic muscle group. It will be difficult to determine actual strength if the muscle group is hypertonic and evidencing exaggerated stretch reflexes.
6. Compare strength bilaterally.

Grip Strength Dynamometers and Cynamometers

Grip strength dynamometers are hand-held devices which measure grip strength in pounds or grams of force. The individual stands or sits while holding the dynamometer along the side of the body or above the head. The device is then squeezed (isometrically) as hard as possible for several seconds while exhaling. When using a starting position above the head, the dynamometer is brought down to the side as the maximal effort is elicited. This maneuver activates more motor units and thus more strength. Two trials are usually allowed and both hands are tested.

Cynamometers are devices created for those with paresis of the hands. It is a more sensitive device than the hand dynamometer and is designed to accommodate contractures of the hand. The individual squeezes a rubber bulb which comes in several sizes and registers force on a dial. Pinch strength may also be evaluated with this device.

Repetition Maximum (RM) with Weights

Strength may be assessed by the maximal amount of weight that can be lifted for a certain number of repetitions, usually between one to 10 repetitions. It is recommended that a 10-RM be used for strength evaluations in adapted physical education programs. This method is based on DeLorme's Progressive Resistive Exercise technique. The following protocol is used to establish a 10-RM:

Warm up set   10 repetitions at 50% of 10-RM
Practice set   10 repetitions at 75% of 10-RM
Maximal set   10 repetitions at 100% of 10-RM

The purpose of the warm up set is to increase muscle irritability. The second set allows for practice of the lifting technique. The third set is the maximal amount of weight that can be lifted in 10 repetitions or 10-RM.

Example: 10 repetitions at 50 lbs.
10 repetitions at 75 lbs.
10 repetitions at 100 lbs.

Isokinetic Testing

Isokinetic testing allows for assessing muscular strength at a range of movement velocities. This feature is an advantage over istonic devices because some persons with coordination problems may not demonstrate deficits in strength until they are tested at higher speeds. Some examples of isokinetic equipment used for evaluating muscular strength and endurance include the Cybex, Orthotron, and Hydragym. Due to its cost, the Cybex is usually not found within adapted physical education programs. The Orthotron is a less expensive piece of equipment that can be used for both isokinetic testing and training of the upper and lower extremities. Protocol for testing with the Orthotron is provided below.

Test Protocol for the Orthotron:

Warm up
1. Gently stretch muscle groups to be tested (hold for 30 seconds, two times).
2. Allow five to 10 submaximal efforts at each speed to be tested to check proper alignment, individual tolerance, and familiarize the participant with the test requirements.

Positioning and Stabilization
1. Note the height of the dynamometer head. Aligning a joint's axis of rotation with the axis of rotation of the dynamometer head has a significant effect on the accuracy of torque measurement. In the shoulder joint, the axis will change throughout the movement so a compromise must be determined.
2. Note the distance between the seat and the edge of the lever arm.
3. Note the length of the lever arm; i.e., the location of the tibial pad. The tibial pad should be positioned just above the ankle joint.
4. Stabilize the thigh with the strap provided. Have the participant grip the handles and keep the trunk against the seatback.

Test Protocol (see Table 6-2)
1. Record the highest torque achieved (ft. lbs.) at each test speed.
2. To perform an endurance test, use the speed setting of 7. Record the number of repetitions taken to reach one-half of the maximum (beginning) torque.

Table 6-2. *Test Protocol*

Testing Pattern	Strength		Power	
	Test Speed	No. Max Efforts	Test Speed	No. Max Efforts
Shoulder: Ext/Flex Abd/Add	3	3	7	5
Knee: Ext/Flex	3	3	7	5
Ankle: Plantar flex Dorsiflex	2	3	5	5

Programming for Muscular Strength and Endurance

Prior to embarking on any of the training programs described in this chapter, the instructor should check to see that all participants have turned in the paperwork required for entrance into the program. This paperwork should include the medical history and medical release signed by a physician. The instructor should combine this information with that obtained during the assessment to design the individualized exercise prescription. The following section will aid the instructor in selecting appropriate exercises and techniques for the development of muscular strength and endurance.

Techniques in Strength Training

Strength training techniques currently available to adapted physical educators include the following:

1. Active-assistive exercise
2. Active exercise
3. Isometric exercise
4. Manual resistive exercise with a partner
5. Proprioceptive Neuromuscular Facilitation (PNF)
6. Isotonic exercise
7. Isokinetic exercise

The definitions, advantages, and disadvantages of each exercise technique are presented below. The initials in parentheses beside each subheading suggest how the technique can be indicated on the exercise program card.

Active-Assistive Exercise (AA)

Active-assistive exercise is recommended when the agonist muscle group is so weak that it cannot move the limb through the entire range of motion without assistance from another person. The participant should initiate the movement (e.g., elbow flexion), but the assistant helps overcome the "sticking point" (i.e., where weight of the limb and gravity are too great to voluntarily overcome) and takes the limb through the remainder of the range. This type of exercise may be performed in an anti-gravity or gravity-neutralized position. For particular muscle groups, such as the abdominals, eccentric contractions may be indicated when using active-assistive exercise. Muscles can usually accommodate more resistance with an eccentric contraction than a concentric one. For example, if a participant requires a great deal of assistance to perform an abdominal curl, the assistant should bring the participant to the fully curled position, but then allow the participant to lower himself/herself to the mat without help. Once sufficient strength has been achieved with eccentric contractions, the participant should progress to concentric contractions.

Active Exercise (A)

The participant contracts the agonist muscle group (e.g., elbow flexion) through the range of motion without any resistance other than the weight of the limb and gravity. Active exercise can also be performed in an anti-gravity position. When the participant is able to perform one set of 10 repetitions through the entire range of motion, then he/she should progress to some form of resistive exercise.

Resistive Exercise

During resistive exercise, the participant contracts the agonist muscle group through the full range of motion against a given resistance. The amount of resistance and the number of repetitions performed will vary depending on whether the individual is working on strength or endurance.

Types of Resistive Exercise

Isometric Exercise (I)

Isometric exercise involves exerting muscular force against an immovable object, thereby creating a static contraction. It may also be created by simply contracting a muscle group statically. Thus, no movement occurs (i.e., no change in the length of the muscle or joint angle). Although tension and heat are produced, mechanical work does not occur. The force exerted may be submaximal or maximal, depending upon the purpose of the exercise. The advantage of isometric exercise is that it does not require any equipment or space to execute. It is also useful if a contracture exists. The disadvantages of isometric exercise are that: (1) it may raise the blood pressure to high levels; (2) the strength gain is specific to the angle trained at (i.e., not much strength gain for the remaining range of motion except 15 degrees to either side of the training angle); and (3) the amount of transfer to functional activities is questionable. Isometric exercise is usually performed in sets of 10 repetitions. Each contraction is held for approximately five to 10 seconds.

Manual Resistive Exercise (MR)

In manual resistive exercise, the participant contracts the agonist muscle group through the range of motion against a resistance applied by the assistant. This effort may be maximal or submaximal, and be performed concentrically or eccentrically. It is usually performed in sets of 10 repetitions or one continuous set to fatigue. The exercise should be performed rhythmically, and if desired, resistance can be applied in both directions or movement (e.g., flexion and extension). The advantages of MR are that: (1) it requires no equipment or space; (2) it is accommodating to the participant's strength levels; and (3) it is useful when contractures prevent positioning on equipment. Manual resistive exercise is typically performed with single joint movements in one plane only (e.g., elbow flexion, sagittal plane); therefore, it does not simulate the majority of functional human movement. Specific MR exercises may be found under "Exercises for Developing Strength and Endurance" in this chapter.

Proprioceptive Neuromuscular Facilitation (PNF)

PNF is a group of relaxation and strengthening techniques used to rehabilitate neuromuscular deficiencies. It refers to the facilitation of neuromuscular activity by stimulating proprioceptive sensory input which regulates muscle function, joint movement, locomotion, posture, and body space. For example, PNF takes advantage of the neuromuscular phenomena of autogenic inhibition, reciprocal inhibition, and stretch reflex to faciliate voluntary movement and relaxation. Proprioceptors include the muscle spindle, Golgi Tendon Organ, and joint receptors. However, PNF takes advantage of all the senses. Additional facilitation is achieved through use of the eyes (e.g., individual observes movement), ears (e.g., individual receives commands; posture regulated by the inner ear), and the exteroceptors of the skin (e.g., tactile input by the therapist). Treatments are directed toward the improvement of the individual's ability to perform functional activities.

The patterns of motion utilized in PNF follow spiral/diagonal pathways (e.g., shoulder flexion-adduction-internal rotation) to make total use of the muscles. The inclusion of rotation adds synergistic muscles to the movement. PNF should only be performed through the pain-free range of motion.

PNF techniques are based upon many of Sherrington's principles (1947): (1) facilitating strong components before weak; (2) applying maximal resistance (irradiation); and (3) successive induction. It is beyond the scope of this manual to provide a comprehensive explanation of the techniques involved in PNF. It is also a method which requires much experience to be competent. Several textbooks are available at medical book stores that describe the technique in detail.

Technique Components of PNF

Maximal Resistance

Apply an amount of resistance which allows the participant to move rhythmically and pain-free through the range of motion. Work within the participant's existing range. Isometric contractions can also be used.

Pressure/Manual Contact

1. Place hands on participant in direction of desired movement.
2. Do not use a circular grip on the limb. Use even, lumbrical grip: MP flexion, IP extension.
3. Resistance is applied in the exact opposite direction of motion - this guides the participant through the pattern.
4. Use proper body position (assistant should stand as part of the diagonal).
5. Facilitory technique by pressure.

Quick Stretch

1. Facilitory in beginning of pattern because it triggers the stretch reflex of the muscle spindles.
2. Followed by resistance (facilitory).
3. Do not use in painful joints or joint restrictions.

Traction

1. Separation of joint structures.
2. Elongate muscle and joint capsule.
3. Muscles brought to taut position.
4. Used in anti-gravity or flexion patterns.
5. Aids in stabilizing and controlling joint motion.

Approximation

1. Joint compression through long axis of structure.
2. Co-contraction of proximal component.
3. Facilitates extension and postural reflex.
4. Used in extension patterns.
5. Most effective in lower extremities.
6. Can be maintained through the range or applied at the end range.
7. Contraindications: joint disease, osteomyelitis, non-weight bearing joints, fractures, painful joints.

Verbal Stimulation

1. Amount and type depends upon cognitive level.
2. Use simple, concise commands.
3. Use a strong voice to facilitate maximal effort.

Visual Stimulation

Becomes an important modality when tactile sensation and proprioception are deficient. Have participant watch the limb that is being exercised.

Timing

Progress from distal movements to proximal movements or proximal to distal. Stronger muscles cause irradiation to the weaker.

Specific Techniques of PNF

1. Rhythmic Stabilization (R-S). Move joint to the point of limitation. Hold the pattern isometrically and maximally until the participant begins to tire. Change resistance to the antagonist muscle group and hold isometrically. Move to a new point of limitation.
2. Hold-Relax (H-R). See description in Chapter 7.
3. Contract-Relax (C-R). Move joint to point of limitation. Contract isotonically with antagonist muscle group. Move to a new point of limitation. Repeat until no new further range of motion is obtainable.
4. Rhythmic Initiation (R-I). The assistant guides the participant through the pattern until it is learned. Resistance is gradually increased as the pattern is learned.

5. Slow Reversals (S-R). Provide resistance in one diagonal pattern through range of motion and then reverse the pattern to the opposite direction. Perform one set to fatigue.
6. Repeated Contractions (R-C). Provide resistance in one diagonal pattern until a weak point is found in the range. Hold at that point and build up to a maximal isometric contraction. Pull the limb back and move forward again. Repeat several times.

Isotonic Exercise, Progressive Exercise Resistive (PRE)

In isotonic exercise, resistance is provided by a weight such as a dumbbell, pulley, ankle/wrist weight, or weight training machine. Because the resistance remains constant throughout the movement, this form of exercise does not accommodate the changes in strength that occur as the joint angle changes (i.e., a muscle group is strongest at midrange and weaker at the end ranges). Thus, isotonic exercise may be considered submaximal when compared to MR or PNF because it cannot fully accommodate the strongest portion of the range. Some mechanical devices (e.g., Nautilus, Universal Centurion machines) use cams to change the amount of resistance encountered through the range of motion. This type of machine accommodates the muscle capabilities to a much greater degree than the constant resistance provided by a dumbbell or the standard Universal equipment.

Protocols using isotonic exercise vary widely. Progressive Resistance Exercise (PRE) is one technique which has been used extensively in rehabilitation and strength training programs for several decades. De Lorme and Watkins were the first to describe the technique in 1951. PRE constitutes only one aspect of the total rehabilitation program and that is the development of absolute strength. It does not necessarily purport to develop muscular endurance or speed of movement.

PRE relies upon both concentric and eccentric contractions of the muscle as the weight is lifted and lowered. Additional muscles are utilized through static contractions to stabilize skeletal parts while movement is occurring. During the eccentric contraction, the muscle is taken beyond its normal resting length, thus facilitating greater force development than in the proceeding concentric contraction.

To overload the muscle for strength development, PRE prescribes the heaviest load which can be lifted through the range of motion for 10 repetitions (10-RM). This is preceded by two warm up sets of 10 repetitions at submaximal loads. The purpose of the warm up is to increase muscle irritability and to allow practice of the lifting technique. A forth and fifth set at the 10-RM facilitates the development of endurance.

Protocol: Establish 10-RM	**Example**
1st set — 50% of 10-RM	1st set — 6 lbs.
2nd set — 75% of 10-RM	2nd set — 9 lbs.
3rd set — 100% of 10-RM	3rd set — 12 lbs.
4th set — 100% of 10-RM (optional for endurance)	
5th set — 100% of 10-RM (optional for endurance)	The 10-RM must be re-established as strength is gained.

Isokinetic Exercise

The participant contracts the agonist muscle group through the range of motion against a lever of constant speed, thereby achieving a maximal effort at every point in the range. Because it accommodates the strength changes that occur as the joint angle changes, isokinetic exercise theoretically enables one to perform more work than with isotonic methods. Only reciprocal movements with concentric contractions occur with isokinetic exercise. The exerciser does not lift weight but pushes against a lever that moves at a fixed speed in both directions (e.g., flexion/extension). Thus, it allows the instructor to measure strength imbalances about a joint (e.g., knee flexors should be approximately 60% the strength of the knee extensors at slower velocities of movement). Isokinetic devices offer a range of speeds to select for training.

General Guidelines for Adapted Weight Training

When using resistive exercise, the weight training program can be divided into three phases (see Table 6-3). This same protocol can be followed whether using weights or manual resistance. The purpose of Phase I is to: (1) learn the mechanics of the lift; (2) practice the proper breathing pattern; and (3) prevent injury to previously weak and atrophied muscles. Individuals who have not exercised for an extended period of time are especially prone to sudden strains, soreness, or inflammations if they immediately begin a rigorous exercise regime. Phase I involves lifting a set of 15 repetitions at a relatively light poundage. This regime continues for approximately two weeks.

During Phase II, the poundage is increased while repetitions are decreased to between 8 and 12 per set (three set minimum). It is advisable to establish a 10-RM at this time and follow the PRE protocol (see PRE earlier in this chapter). **Always have your participants perform at least one warm-up set prior to a 10-RM!** If the participant can lift the weight for more than 12 repetitions during the final set (i.e., exceeds the 10-RM), then increase the amount of weight on the next exercise day.

If muscular endurance is desired, the participant can proceed to Phase III. Rather than increasing the amount of weight lifted, the repetitions are increased to between 12 and 20. These repetitions may be performed in sets of three. A poundage should be selected that allows only the desired number of repetitions to be completed. If manual resistance or PNF is used, one continuous set to fatigue may be used. For many persons who use manual wheelchairs, the development of muscular endurance may be more important than absolute strength.

Table 6-3. *Phases of a Strength/Endurance Program*

	Phase I	Phase II	Phase III
Sets	1-2	3	3
Reps	15	8-12	12-20
Load	Light	Moderate/Heavy	Moderate
Minimum Duration	2 weeks	6-8 weeks	Indefinite
Purpose	Practice	Strength	Endurance

Guidelines for Conducting a Safe and Beneficial Strength Program

1. Keep accurate, daily records of your participant's performance. This procedure includes recording the date, poundage used, and the number of sets and repetitions performed.

2. Retest every few weeks to reestablish the 10-RM.

3. Supervise with a spotter (assistant) when a participant is lifting weights - no matter how light the poundage!

4. Alternate upper and lower body exercises so no two consecutive exercises involve the same prime mover.

5. Perform exercises which involve larger muscle groups first. For example, perform shoulder strengthening exercises before wrist exercises.

6. Allow sufficient recovery time between sets (usually several minutes), especially for those with degenerative neuromuscular conditions. For highly fit athletes, the rest period can be reduced as strength and endurance improve.

7. Lift no more than every other day with the same strength training routine.

8. Perform each repetition rhythmically and without a pause at the beginning or end of the range of motion.

9. Precede maximal lifts with a warm up set.

10. FOLLOW A WEIGHT LIFTING SESSION WITH FLEXIBILITY EXERCISES TO PREVENT ADAPTIVE SHORTENING FROM OCCURRING. Muscles retain some residual tension or contraction after strenuous exercise and should be brought back to their original to resting length.

11. Maintain good muscular balance by strengthening opposing muscle groups, unless an imbalance already exists.

12. Breathe properly during weight lifting. Exhale on effort. Inhale when lowering weight.

13. Have the participant watch himself/herself perform the movement. Vision is especially important when deficiencies in proprioception exist.

14. Begin an exercise from a position of "on stretch" and then move into a concentric contraction. This facilitates the intensity of the contraction.

15. Develop strength before endurance in a weight training program.

16. Increase the difficulty of a weight training program by increasing resistance, repetitions, or number of sets. Remember - using too heavy of a weight may cause improper form (leading to injury) and should be avoided.

Interpreting the Exercise Program Card

As was previously mentioned in Chapter 1, the exercise program card for weight training should contain the following information: (1) name; (2) dates for every day the participant exercised in the program; (3) names of exercises and prescription; (4) daily recording of sets, repetitions, and loads lifted; (5) disabilities; (6) contraindications; and (7) effects of any medications. The assistant should never change the exercise program card without approval from the instructor. The assistant should make sure the card is filled out completely and dated each day. In addition, a card for "progress notes" can be attached to the exercise program card to allow for recording of qualitative information (e.g., pain occurring during a particular exercise).

Consistent terminology should be used when describing exercises on the program card. This allows for interchanging of assistants without confusion. Exercises should be named according to the following system:

1. **Anatomical movement**: For single joint movements, write the name of the joint and its anatomical movement. The body position will also have to be indicated. For example: Elbow flexion - sitting. All anatomical movement and body positions are described in Chapter 2.
2. **Approved vernacular**: If multi-joint movement is involved in performing the exercise, then use an approved vernacular. These types of exercises are described later in this chapter. For example: Lat Pull, Bench Press.
3. **Abbreviated description**: If the exercise has been modified for the participant or there is no accepted name for it, a brief description can be written in.

A prescription should accompany the name of the exercise and body position. Sets and repetitions may be prescribed in the following manner, respectively: 3 X 10 This formula is interpreted as three sets of 10 repetitions. The exercise program card should have boxes which allow for recording the number of sets, repetitions, and weight that were lifted on a given day. If manual resistance is to be used in place of weights, then "MR" can be indicated by the exercise on the card. In exercise #1 on the sample card, the prescription is interpreted as one set of 10 repetitions for right knee flexion in the prone position, using manual resistance with an assistant. An example of a sample program exercise card is as follows;

Sample Program Exercise Card

		date	date	date	
1. (R)	MR 1 • 10 knee flexion-prone				
2.	3 • 10 bench press				

Exercises for Developing Muscular Strength and Endurance

The exercises described in this section can be performed with the following strength training techniques: active-assistive, active, isometric, manual resistive, and isotonic (PRE). The photos illustrate some active, isometric, manual resistive, and isotonic techniques (the latter using using pulleys and free weights). The reader is referred to Chapter 2 for a listing of muscles which are strengthened in single joint, anatomical movements. For multi-joint exercises, the prime movers have been identified in this chapter.

This list is not meant to be inclusive of all possible strength exercises available to adapted physical educators. Many of the manual resistive and free weight exercises in this section can be performed in body positions other than the ones presented here. Additionally, many of these exercises can be performed in the pool, using the water as the resistive medium. The use of a kickboard with the shoulder exercises adds additional resistance.

Action

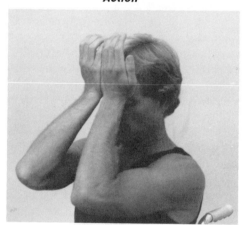

Cervical Flexion

Position: Sitting or standing

Action: Keep head in anatomical position. Place palms on forehead. Press forehead isometrically into palms, attempting to flex neck. Hold each repetition (rep) for five seconds.

Action

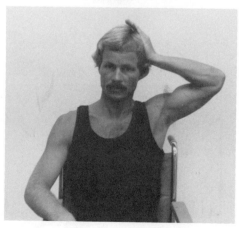

Cervical Rotation

Position: Sitting or Standing

Action: Keep head in anatomical position. Place left hand on left, lateral aspect of head. Attempt to rotate head to left, creating an isometric contraction. Hold each rep five seconds. Repeat with right hand to right, lateral aspect of head.

Shoulder Girdle Elevation

Position: Sitting (a & b), Standing (b)

Action:
  a. Assistant places hands on acromion processes of participant and attempts to keep shoulders depressed. Participant attempts to elevate shoulders up to ears.
  b. Participant holds dumbbells in each hand and attempts to elevate shoulders up to ears.

Action (a)

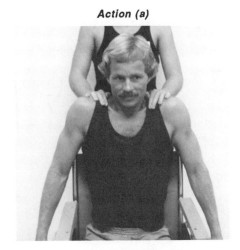

Shoulder Flexion

Position: Sitting (a, b & c), Standing (c)

Action:
  a. Participant flexes elbow to 90 degrees. Assistant places one hand on superior aspect of shoulder to stabilize and other hand on anterior aspect of upper arm. Participant flexes shoulder against resistance provided by assistant. Repeat to other side.
  b. Face sideways to pulley. Grasp lower pulley with one hand. Keeping the arm straight, pull up and across the front of the body, flexing and horizontally adducting at the shoulder. Repeat to other side. For pure shoulder flexion, face away from pulley and raise arm straight out in front of body.
  c. Hold dumbbell in hand. Keeping arm straight, flex at shoulder, bringing weight out in front of body. Repeat to other side.

Action (a)

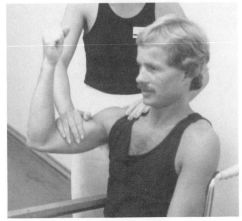

Action (b)

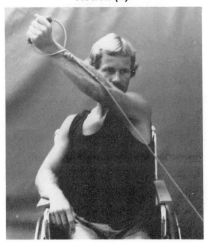

Shoulder Abduction (to 90 degrees)

Position: Sitting (a, b, & c), Standing (c)

Action:
  a. Participant flexes elbows. Assistant places hand on lateral aspect of arm, proximal to elbow. Participant abducts shoulder against assistant's resistance.
  b. Participant faces sideways to low pulley. Keeping arm straight, lower pulley is brought up by abducting shoulder. Repeat to other side. Alternative: Grasp pulley handle with hand farthest from low wall pulley, palm in a supinated position, elbow extended. Abduct arm to 90°.
  c. Participant holds dumbbell in each hand and abducts both shoulders, bringing weight above shoulders.

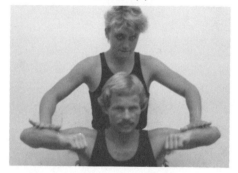
Action (a)

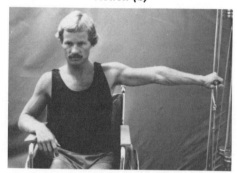
Action (b)

Shoulder Extension/ Hyperextension

Position: Sitting (a & b), Standing (b)

Action:
  a. Participant flexes elbow to 90°. Assistant places one hand on superior aspect on shoulder and other on posterior aspect of arm, proximal to elbow. Student attempts to extend/hyperextend shoulder against resistance. Repeat to other side.
  b. Facing high pulley and keeping the arm straight, participant grasps upper pulley (palm facing backwards) and extends/hyperextends shoulder. Repeat to other side.

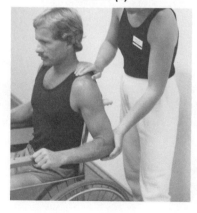
Action (a)

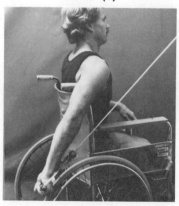
Action (b)

Upright Rows (elbow flexion & shoulder abduction)

Muscles: Trapezius, Deltoids, Biceps

Position: Sitting (a), Standing (b)

Action:
   a. Face pulleys and grasp lower handles. Pull and bring hands up to chin, flexing at the elbows.
   b. Hold barbell in both hands. Bring bar up to chin. A cane with a sand weight attached may be substituted for the barbell.

Shoulder Horizontal Abduction

Position: Sitting (a & b), Standing (b), Prone on a low bench (c)

Action:
   a. Participant flexes elbows and horizontally adducts shoulders. Assistant places hands on posterior aspect of arm, proximal to elbow. Participant horizontally adducts shoulders against resistance.
   b. Face pulleys and grasp upper handles. Pull handles out to sides with slightly flexed elbows. Attempt to bring hands behind back. Alternative: Face sideways and grasp with farthest hand, raise arm to shoulder level and pull horizontally.
   c. Hold dumbbell in each hand and horizontally abduct shoulders, keeping elbow slightly flexed. Attempt to bring hands behind back.

Action (a)

Action (b)

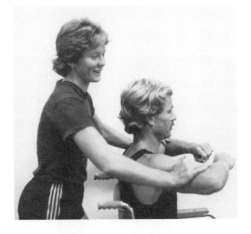

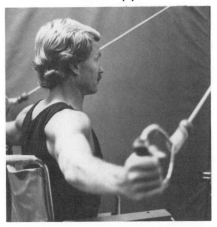

Shoulder Horizontal Adduction

Position: Sitting (a & b), Standing (b), Supine on a low bench (c)

Action:
   a. Participant flexes elbows and abducts shoulders. Assistant places hands on anterior aspect of upper arms. Participant horizontally adducts shoulders against resistance.
   b. Participant faces sideways to pulleys, grasping the upper handles. Keeping the elbow slightly flexed, the handle is brought horizontally across the front of the body. Repeat to other side.
   c. Holding a dumbbell in each hand, participant keeps elbows slightly flexed and horizontally adducts shoulders, bringing the weight out in front of the body.

Action (a)

Action (b)

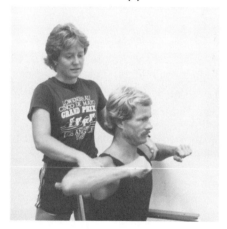

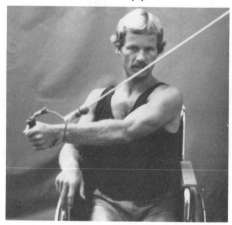

Pull-Over

Muscles: Pectoralis Major, Triceps

Position: Supine hook-lying

Action: Participant grasps one dumbbell with both hands at the midline. Keeping arms slightly flexed at the elbows, the dumbbell is brought up and behind the head.

Bench Press

Muscles: Pectorals, Deltoids, Triceps

Position: Supine hook-lying on bench (a) or mat (b)

Action:
   a. Keep feet on bench. Grasp handles, keeping them as close as possible to the long axis of forearm. Press weight up and exhale simultaneously.
   b. Hold dumbbell in each hand, keeping forearms pronated. Shoulders are abducted. Press the weight upward and exhale until elbows are extended.

Shoulder Adduction

Position: Sitting (a & b), Standing (b)

Action:
   a. Participant abducts shoulders and flexes elbows. Assistant places hands on medial aspect of arm, proximal to elbow. Participant adducts shoulders against resistance.
   b. Face sideways to pulleys. Grasp the upper handle and pull down to side, adducting shoulder. Keep arm straight. Repeat to other side.

Action (a)

Action (b)

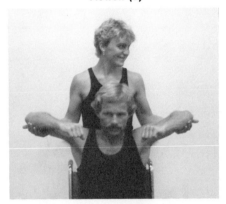

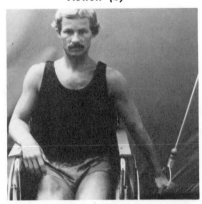

Lat Pull Down

Muscles: Latissimus Dorsi, Trapezius, Teres Major, Rhomboids Minor, Deltoids, Biceps and Brachialis, Triceps, Pectorals

Position: Sitting or kneeling, facing apparatus

Action: Participant should be positioned directly under bar. Grasp bar with a wide grip and pull down to back of neck or front to sternum.

Shoulder External Rotation

Position: Supine hook-lying (a), Prone on a table(b)

Action:
a. Participant flexes elbow and abducts shoulder. Assistant places one hand on dorsum of hand and other stabilizes the elbow. Participant externally rotates shoulder against resistance. Repeat to other side.
b. Hold dumbbell in one hand with shoulder abducted and elbow flexed. Externally rotate shoulder slowly. Repeat to other side.

Action (a)

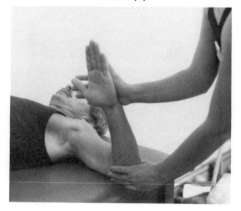

Action (b)

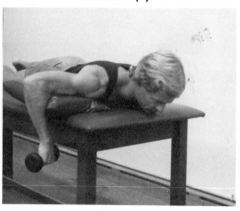

Action

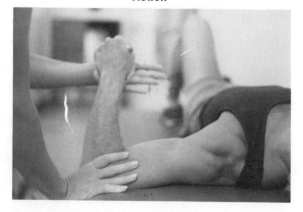

Shoulder Internal Rotation

Position: Supine hook-lying

Action: Participant flexes elbow and abducts shoulder. Assistant places one hand on palmar surface and stabilizes the elbow with the other. Participant internally rotates against resistance. Repeat to other side.

Elbow Flexion

Position: Sitting (a, b & c), Standing (c)

Action:
   a. Assistant places one hand against medial side of arm, proximal to wrist, while other hand stabilizes the elbow. Participant flexes elbow against resistance. Repeat to other side.
   b. Facing pulley, participant grasps lower handle and stabilizes elbow on armrest. Participant then brings handle up, flexing at elbow. Repeat to other side.
   c. Hold dumbell in hand. Flex at elbow, bringing hand up to shoulder level.

Action (a)

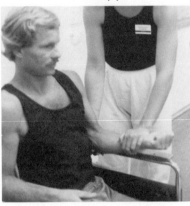

Action (b)

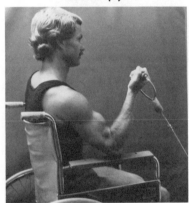

Elbow Extension

Position: Supine hook-lying (a), Sitting or Standing (b & d), Long sitting (c)

Action:
   a. Participant flexes elbow. Assistant stabilizes elbow with one hand and places the other on lateral aspect of arm at wrist joint. Participant extends elbow against resistance. Repeat to other side.
   b. Face away from pulley. Grasping the upper handles, extend elbow (elbow should be stabilized on armrest or participant can use other arm to do this). Repeat to other side.
   c. Grasping push up blocks, participant extends elbows, raising buttocks off the mat.
   d. Use lat pull bar. Standing or sitting slightly behind bar, grasp handles and pull bar down until elbows are touching sides of trunk. Keep elbows into sides and extend at the elbows only.

Action (a)

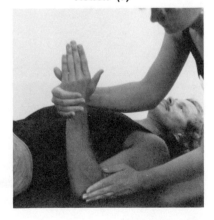

Elbow Extension (continued)

Action (b)

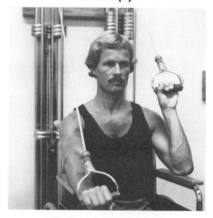

Action (c)

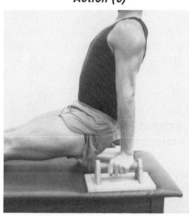

Action

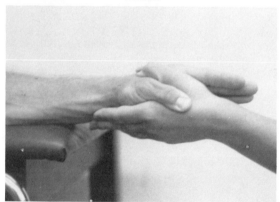

Forearm Pronation

Position: Sitting

Action: Assistant shakes hands with participant, keeping thumb off dorsum of participant's hand. Forearm should be stabilized on a padded table. Participant pronates forearm against resistance. Repeat to other side.

Action

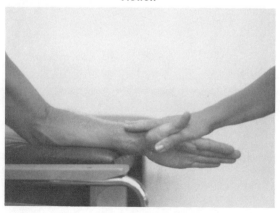

Forearm Supination

Position: Sitting

Action: Assistant places one hand on dorsum of participant's hand Participant's forearm should be stabilized on padded table. Participant supinates forearm against resistance. Repeat to other side.

Wrist Flexion

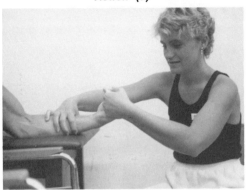

Action (a)

Position: Sitting

Action:
a. Assistant places one hand in palm of participant while stabilizing forearm with other hand. Participant flexes wrist against resistance. Repeat to other side.
b. Hold dumbbell in hand with wrist extended over edge of table. Flex wrist up. Repeat to other side.

Wrist Extension

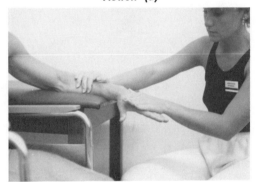

Action (a)

Position: Sitting

Action:
a. Assistant places one hand on dorsum of participant's hand while stabilizing the forearm with the other. Participant tends wrist against resistance. Repeat to other side.
b. Hold dumbbell in hand, palm down, with wrist extended over side of table. Extend wrist up. Repeat to other side.

Thumb and Finger Flexion, Pinch

Position: Sitting

Action: Use theraplast (silly putty) to squeeze with thumb and fingers simultaneously. Place a ball between thumb, index, and middle fingers - pinch.

Spinal Flexion (abdominal curls)

Position: Supine hook-lying (a, b, & c), Sitting (d)

Action:
   a. Flex hips and knees 90 degrees with the lower legs supported by a low bench. Place hands across chest. Slowly curl one-third of distance up (scapula should clear ground) and lower. May also slowly twist right and left.
   b. Reach left arm toward right knee. Contract abdominals, keeping low back pressed to floor.
   c. Place hands under hips. Bring knees to chest, lifting hips off mat.
   d. Face away from pulley, grasping upper handles. Flex spine forward.

Action (a)

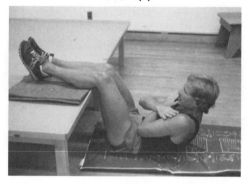

Action (b)

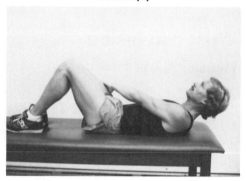

Action (c)

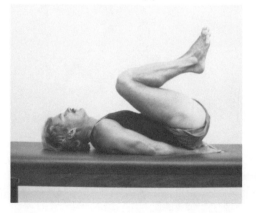

Action (d)

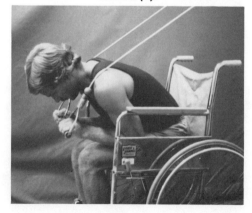

Spinal Extension

Position: Sitting (a & b), Prone on mat (c)

Action:
  a. Assistant places hands on participant's scapula. Participant flexes forward as far as possible and then extends spine against resistance.
  b. Face pulleys and grasp lower handles. Extend spine.
  c. With shoulders abducted, rotate thumbs up toward the ceiling, raise upper trunk off mat, and pinch shoulder blades together. Hold for five seconds.

Action (a)

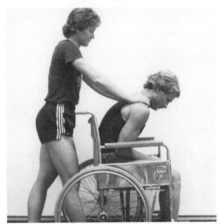

Action (b)

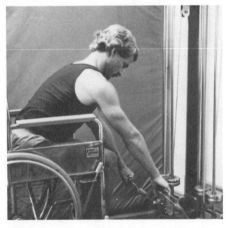

Action (c)

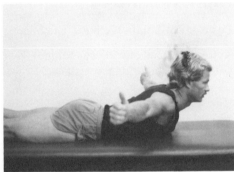

When doing this extension, you may want to place a small pillow under the hips to protect the lower back.

Lateral Flexion

Position: Sitting

Action: Face sideways to pulley. Grasping lower handles, laterally flex spine over armrest. Repeat to other side.

Action

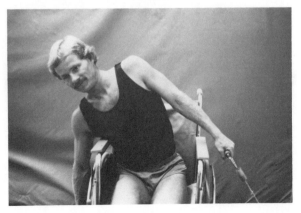

Action

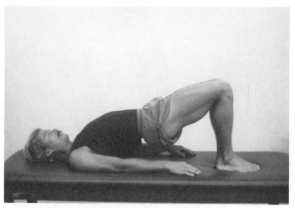

Hip Hikers or Bridges (lumbar extension, hip extension)

Position: Supine hook-lying

Action: Place feet and knees together. Elevate hip off mat. Hold five seconds.

Hip Extension

Position: 4-point on elbows and knees

Action: Extend one leg out behind. Extend up and down at hip. Using an ankle weight will provide additional resistance. Repeat to other side.

Action

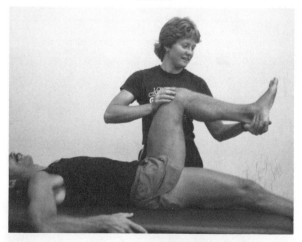

Hip Flexion

Position: Supine

Action: Assistant places one hand on anterior aspect of leg, proximal to knee. The other hand may need to stabilize the foot. Participant flexes hip against resistance. Repeat to other side.

Hip Adduction

Position: Supine (a), Side-lying (b), Standing (c)

Action:
  a. Assistant places one hand against medial aspect of knee and the other against the medial aspect of the ankle. Keeping the leg extended, participant adducts hip against resistance. Repeat to other side.
  b. Prop up on elbow and place superior leg in front, flexing at the knee. Using an ankle weight, adduct hip of lower leg, keeping knee extended. Repeat to the other side.
  c. Face sideways to pulleys and attach closest ankle to lower handles. Adduct hip. Repeat to other side.

Action (a)

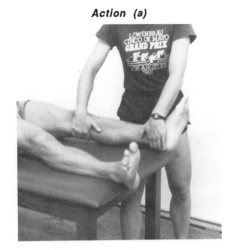

Hip Abduction

Position: Supine (a), Side-lying (b), Standing (c)

Action:
  a. Assistant places one hand on lateral aspect of knee and the other against the lateral aspect of ankle. Keeping the leg extended, participant abducts hip against resistance. Repeat to other side.
  b. Using an ankle weight, participant abducts hip, keeping knee extended and leg rotated inward. Repeat to other side.
  c. Face sideways to pulleys and attach farthest ankle to lower handles. Abduct hip. Repeat to other side.

Action (a)

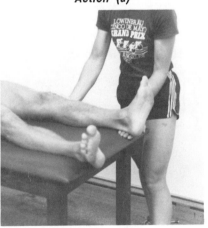

Hip Internal Rotation

Position: Supine

Action: Assistant places one hand on medial aspect of knee and the other on the medial aspect of foot. Participant internally rotates leg against resistance. Repeat to other side.

Action

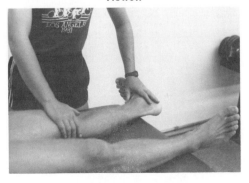

Action

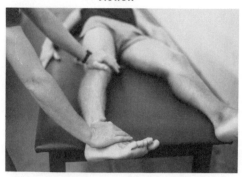

Hip External Rotation

Position: Supine

Action: Assistant places one hand on lateral aspect of knee and the other on the lateral aspect of foot. Participant externally rotates leg against resistance. Repeat to other side.

Leg Press

Muscles: Quadriceps, Gluteus Maximus

Position: Long sitting on Universal leg press

Action: Extend at the hip and knee. BE SURE **NOT** TO LOCK OR HYPEREXTEND THE KNEE DURING THIS EXERCISE!

Knee Extension

Position: Sitting (a & c), Long sitting on the elbows (b)

Action:
   a. Participant sits on plinth with knees over edge. Assistant places one hand on dorsal surface of foot and the other on the medial side of heel. Participant extends knee against resistance. Repeat to other side.
   b. Used in conjunction with a quad board and ankle weight. Dorsiflex ankle and extend knee, holding for five seconds. Emphasis should be on the vastus medialis. Quad board is adjusted to allowable range of motion.
   c. Knee extension may also be performed on a Universal machine.

Action (a)

Action (b)

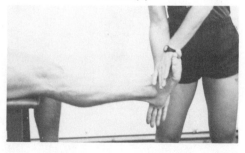

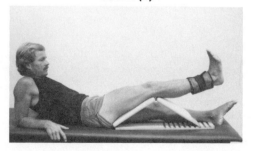

Knee Flexion

Position: Prone

Action:

  a. Assistant places both hands on the posterior aspect of the lower legs, proximal to the ankle joint. Participant flexes knees against resistance.

  b. Universal knee flexion machine. Flex knees, keeping pelvis flat on the bench.

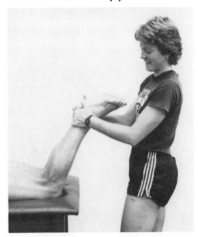

Action (a)

Dorsiflexion

Position: Long sitting

Action: Assistant places one hand on dorsal aspect of foot, proximal to the metatarsophalangeal joints. Participant dorsiflexes the foot against resistance, extending the toes as well. Repeat to other side.

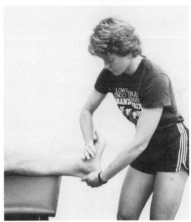

Action

Plantar Flexion

Position: Prone (a), Standing (b), Long sitting (c)

Action:

  a. Assistant places hands on the plantar surface of the foot. Participant plantar flexes foot against resistance. Repeat to other side.

  b. Standing on stairs with the heels off, plantar flex the ankles, raising the feet up and down.

  c. Universal machine (leg press). Keeping the knees extended (with slight flexion), plantar flex the ankles on the foot pedals.

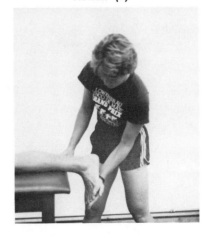

Action (a)

Action (a)

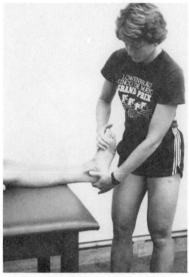

Inversion

Position: Long sitting (a), Sitting (b)

Action:
    a. Assistant places one hand against first metatarsal head. Participant inverts foot against resistance. Repeat to other side.
    b. Place a towel underneath feet. Invert feet together, sweeping towel toward middle. Weights can be placed at the ends of the towel to increase resistance.

Action (a)

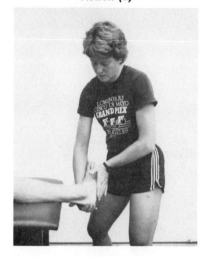

Eversion

Position: Long sitting (a), Sitting (b)

Action:
    a. Assistant places one hand against the fifth metatarsal head. Participant everts foot against resistance. Repeat to other side.
    b. Place a bunched towel underneath feet. Evert feet together, straightening towel out. Weights can be placed at ends of towel to increase resistance.

Study Questions / Learning Activities

1. Differentiate between muscular strength and endurance.

2. Discuss the advantages and disadvantages of the resistive forms of strength techniques.

3. Outline the muscle gradations and criteria for the Manual Muscle Test.

4. Describe the protocol for progressive resistive exercise.

5. Outline the phases of a strength training program.

6. Select an anatomical movement for the shoulder, elbow, hip, and knee. With a partner, demonstrate active-assistive, active, isometric, manual resistive, and isotonic techniques for each movement.

7. Devise a complete strength training program for yourself that includes all major muscle groups. Indicate the order of exercises in your workout.

8. Devise a complete upper body strength training program for a person using a wheelchair (complete spinal cord injury at thoracic nerve root 10 - see Chapter 13). Indicate the order of exercises in the workout, as well as which muscle groups are involved with each exercise.

References

Chawla, J. C., Bar, D., Creber, I., Price, J., & Andrew, B. (1980). Techniques for improving the strength and fitness of spinal cord injured patients. *Paraplegia, 17*, 185-190.

Daniels, L., & Worthingham, C. (1972). *Muscle testing.* Philadelphia: W. B. Saunders.

Davis, G. M., Shephard, R. J., & Jackson, R. W. (1981). Cardio-respiratory fitness and muscular strength in the lower-limb disabled. *Canadian Journal of Applied Sport Sciences, 6*(4), 159-165.

Haskins, M. (1972). *Evaluation in physical education.* Dubuque: W. C. Brown.

Hoppenfeld, S. (1976). *Physical examination of the spine and extremities.* New York: Appleton-Century Crofts.

Knott, M., & Voss, D. E. (1956). *Proprioceptive neuromuscular facilitation. Patterns and techniques.* New York: Hoeber-Harper.

Knutsson, E. (1973). Physical therapy techniques in the control of spasticity. *Scandanavian Journal of Rehabilitative Medicine, 5*, 167-169.

Sharkey, B. J. (1979). *Physiology of fitness. Prescribing exercise for fitness, weight control, and health.* Campaign, Illinois: Human Kinetics.

Sherrill, C. (1986). *Adapted physical education and recreation* (3rd ed.). Dubuque: William C. Brown.

CHAPTER 7

Assessment and Programming for Flexibility

Assessment of Flexibility

Both active and passive range of motion (ROM) tests should be utilized when determining limitations in flexibility. Active ROM tests are performed with the participant actively contracting muscles to take the joint through the full range of motion. Passive ROM testing utilizes an assistant to take the limb through the range and is conducted when the participant has difficulty completing the movement due to lack of strength and/or coordination. In general, if a participant can move a limb through the normal range of motion actively, then a passive ROM test is not required (Hoppenfeld, 1976). Passive ROM is typically greater than active ROM.

The following section will present only active ROM tests. Normal values are usually recorded on the evaluation sheet as "WNL" (Within Normal Limits), while limitations are recorded as "LOM" (Limitation of Motion). Always test ROM bilaterally for comparison (i.e., the ROM for the non-involved joint can be used as the standard for evaluating the LOM in the involved joint). The positions for passive ROM testing can be found under Passive Flexibility Exercises later on in this chaper.

Active Range of Motion Tests (Hoppenfeld, 1976)

Finger Flexion and Extension (metacarpophalangeal joint)

Finger

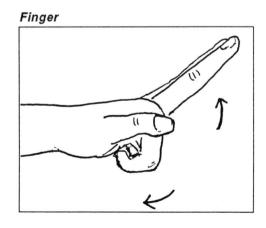

Make a tight fist, then extend the fingers. The fingers should completely close into the palm for flexion (90 degrees) and extend even with or beyond the dorsum of the hand for normal extension (45 degrees). Note whether the fingers work in unison (see illustration).

Wrist

Elbow

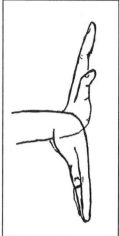
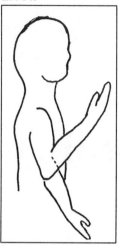

Wrist Flexion and Extension

With extended fingers, flex and extend the wrist. Normal range of motion is approximately 80 degrees for wrist flexion and 70 degrees for wrist extension.

Elbow Flexion and Extension

Beginning in anatomical position, flex the elbow and touch the front of the shoulder with the hand. Normal range of motion is approximately 150 degrees for elbow flexion and zero degrees for elbow extension.

Forearm

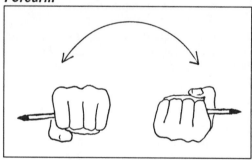

Forearm Supination and Pronation

Flex the elbows and hold them into the sides of the body. Hold a pencil, making a fist with the forearm pronated (palm facing down). Supinate the forearm as far as possible (palm facing up). Normal range of motion is approximately 90 degrees for both pronation and supination.

Shoulder

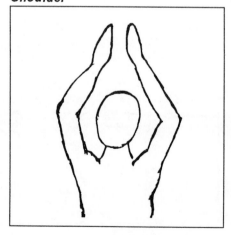

Shoulder Abduction

With extended elbows, abduct the arms to 90 degrees. At 90 degrees, turn palms up, and continue abduction until the palms come together overhead at 180 degrees.

Shoulder External Rotation and Abduction (Apley Scratch Test)

Reach with one hand and touch superior medial angle of the opposite scapula.

Shoulder

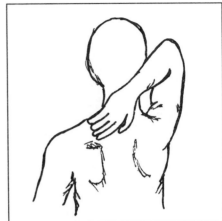

Shoulder Internal Rotation and Adduction

a. Reach behind with one hand touch the inferior angle of the opposite scapula.
b. Reach in front and touch one hand to the opposite shoulder.

Shoulder (a)

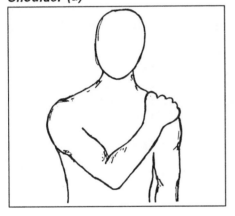

Shoulder (b)

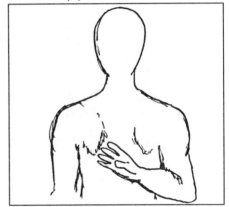

Spinal Flexion (sit-and-reach)

Use the sit-and-reach box. Assume a long sitting position with bare feet against the sit-and-reach box. Place one hand on top of the other (middle fingers even), keep the trunk erect (do not round back and shoulders), reach forward as far as possible by bending at the hip, and hold for 10 seconds (allow one warm up trial). Using zero as the point equivalent for reaching the toes, note the number of plus inches beyond the toes or minus inches below the toes.

Spinal

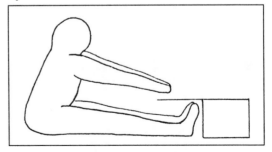

Hip (a)

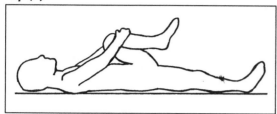

Hip (b)

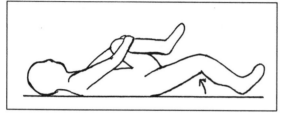

Hip Flexion (Thomas Test)

a. Assume a supine position on a table or mat. Flex the hip, bringing the knee up to the chest. The anterior aspect of the thigh should make contact with the abdomen. Then assess ROM in the other leg. With normal ROM, the other leg (hip) should remain extended and on the table.

b. If the straight leg is not able to extend fully, a hip flexion contracture exists. Estimate the angle between the thigh and the table at the point of greatest extension.

Plantarflexion, Dorsiflexion, Inversion, Eversion (from a standing or sitting position)

a. **Plantarflexion:** bring the heels off the floor 50 degrees.
b. **Dorsiflexion:** bring the toes off the floor 20 degrees.
c. **Inversion:** bring the medial borders of the feet off the floor 5 degrees.
d. **Eversion:** bring the lateral borders of the feet off the floor 5 degrees.

Plantarflexion

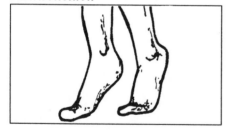

Dorsiflexion

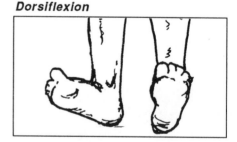

Inversion

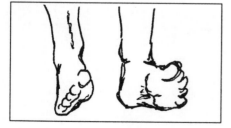

Eversion

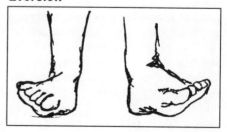

Programming for Flexibility

Optimal Conditions for Eliciting a Stretch

Connective tissue displays both properties of elasticity (rebound to original length) and plasticity (permanent deformation). To increase flexibility, it is important to affect the plastic property of connective tissue. The optimal conditions for achieving a permanent increase in flexibility include the following:

Engage in Warm Up Prior to Stretching

Increasing tissue temperature will facilitate the viscous (plastic) property of connective tissue, resulting in a greater elongation or stretch. In other words, a warm muscle will stretch farther than a cold one! Warm up may include easy laps around the track until a sweat is broken (5-10 minutes). The same result may be achieved by performing calisthenics in place.

Do Not Apply Too Much Force to the Stretch

Lower amounts of force induce less injury and tearing to connective tissue than high amounts of force. Vigorous and/or ballistic stretching may cause bleeding in the joint, as well as tearing of soft tissue.

Hold the Stretch for a Sufficient Duration (The Longer The Better)

Although research has not demonstrated what the optimal duration for a stretch is, it has been agreed that longer durations will produce better results. For purposes of this manual, it is suggested that each stretch be held for a duration of 30-60 seconds. If executed properly, discomfort felt due to stretching will diminish the longer the stretch is held.

Stretching Should Always Be Performed Through the Pain-Free Range of Motion

Do not perform stretching if pain, infection or edema are present.

Incorporate Stretches at the End of Cool-Down to Prevent Adaptive Shortening and Promote Relaxation of Muscle

Muscle which has been subjected to a vigorous workout will generally be in a contracted state. Performing stretching at the end of the workout will return muscle to its resting length and promote additional elongation of connective tissue.

Stretching Techniques

There are two basic types of stretching techniques: active and passive. Active stretching is performed without assistance, using a volitional muscle contraction to move the joint through the full range of motion. In contrast, passive stretching occurs without any muscle contraction and is performed by an assistant. The range of motion about joint is usually greater in a passive stretch than an active one. PNF (proprioceptive neuromuscular facilitation) Hold-Relax is a technique which utilizes both active and passive stretching.

Active Stretching (Slow Static)

This technique involves slowly stretching a muscle for 30-60 seconds (or longer) by contracting the opposing muscle group. If proper stretching is to be accomplished, the lengthened muscle must be held at the point of limitation with a tension level that does not activate, to any marked extent, the stretch reflex mechanism. After holding the stretch for a period of time, the discomfort of tension should diminish to some degree. At this time, the individual may increase the stretch and establish a new point of limitation. This process can be repeated until no further range of motion is attainable. Over-stretching is recognized by discomfort that becomes greater the longer the stretch is held or when the lengthened muscle quivers or vibrates. Avoid bouncing or ballistic movements.

An active stretching routine for participants in wheelchairs is presented in this chapter. Active stretches for ambulatory participants are not provided; the reader is referred to the comprehensive book by Anderson (1980) which is listed at the end of this chapter.

Passive Stretching

This technique is applied when the individual cannot perform an active stretch. It is performed by the assistant and involves ranging every affected joint to prevent contractures from developing through disuse. The assistant moves each joint slowly through the PERMISSIBLE range of motion, using one hand to stabilize the body while the other moves the limb. Hold at the point of limitation for 30-60 seconds. Prolonged, moderate stretching is more effective than momentary, vigorous stretching. Two to five repetitions are usually sufficient for passive range of motion.

PNF (proprioceptive neuromuscular facilitation) Hold-Relax

PNF hold-relax is a relaxation/lengthening technique in which the individual isometrically and maximally contracts a muscle group prior to stretching it to a new point of limitation. The contraction is held for six seconds. When the maximal number of motor units are contracting simultaneously, the Golgi Tendon Organs within that muscle will fire, causing the muscle to relax. This phenomenon is known as autogenic inhibition. During this post-contraction depression, lasting for about six seconds, the Golgi Tendon Organs override the reflex activity of the muscle spindles. The individual or assistant then moves the limb to a new point of limitation. The sequence is repeated until no new further range of motion is obtainable. This technique may be performed with single joint movements, or more ideally, in the spiral/diagonal PNF patterns.

Hold-Relax Sequence:

1. The assistant (passively) or the participant (actively) moves the limb to the point of limitation. Active movement should be encouraged whenever possible. The participant then isometrically and maximally contracts the muscle on stretch against a resistance provided by the assistant for SIX SECONDS. This is the HOLD period of the technique and the limb should not be allowed to move. The maximal contraction should be brought on gradually, not suddenly.
2. The participant then relaxes the stretched muscle and moves the limb to a new point of limitation either actively or passively with help of the assistant This relaxation period for the stretched muscle should last SIX SECONDS. Repeat the sequence of holds and relaxations until no further range of motion is obtained.

Contraindications for Performing Stretching

1. Infections about a joint.
2. Exacerbations (attacks) of inflammatory disease, especially when pain is present.
3. Edema - joint capsule is subject to tears.
4. Functional contractures (e.g., finger flexors, elbow flexors, and pronators may actually assist the participant to pull objects toward him/her).
5. VIGOROUS STRETCHING OF CONTRACTURES. This technique may cause bleeding in the joint. It is the role of the physical therapist, not the adapted physical educator, to improve range of motion in severe contractures.

Performance Requirements for Stretching Techniques

1. Know the anatomical motions that occur at each joint (see Chapter 2).
2. Stabilize the extremities at the joint; for example, at the elbow or wrist. For someone with a painful joint, such as in arthritis, support the extremity in the muscular area.
3. Try to avoid touching the muscle or tendons being stretched as this may trigger unwanted reflex activity.
4. Stretch in opposition to the line of pull of muscle.
5. Use a firm but comfortable grip.

6. Perform motions slowly and smoothly.
7. Do not exceed the participant's existing range of motion, especially in the case of paralyzed limbs. Movements should not be forceful.
8. Never force a stretch if spasticity occurs. Stop applying force and hold the limb or return to the starting position. When the spasticity has subsided, proceed again more slowly and smoothly.
9. Remember, two-jointed muscles need a two-jointed stretch (e.g., hamstrings).

Designating Stretching Exercises on the Program Card

Designate the stretching exercise by using anatomical movement (e.g., shoulder flexion) or an approved vernacular. In addition, indicate body position (e.g., sitting), technique to be used (e.g., A-ROM, P-ROM, PNF Hold-Relax), and quantity to be performed (e.g., 2 * 30 seconds). Assistants should daily record quantity performed.

Passive Flexibility Exercises

Shoulder and Elbow Joint Exercises (1-6)

1. With participant positioned prone, assistant places hands on either side of shoulder and lifts shoulder off of mat, as if bringing the shoulder blades together.

2. With participant supine, assistant places one hand in palm and the other hand on posterior aspect of upper arm. Flex shoulder to end range.

Exercise 1

Exercise 2

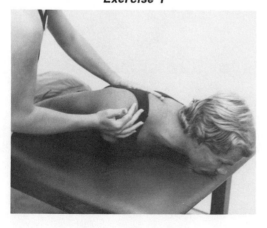
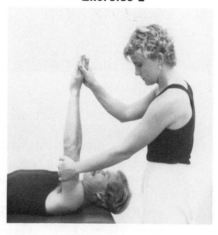

Exercise 3

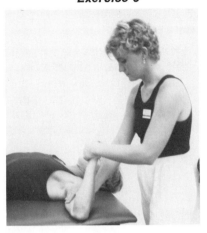

3. With participant supine, shoulder abducted, and elbow flexed, assistant places one hand in palm while the other hand stabilizes upper arm. Externally rotate arm to end range.

Exercise 4

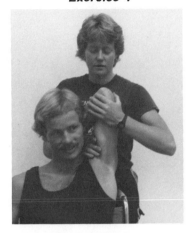

4. With participant sitting, assistant abducts and externally rotates shoulder by placing one hand on posterior aspect of arm, proximal to elbow. The other hand stabilizes at shoulder.

Exercise 5

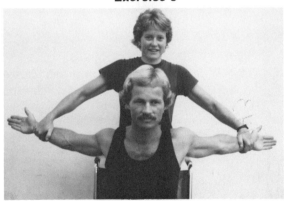

5. With participant sitting, assistant places hands on palmar side of wrists and horizontally abducts arms. The participant's palms should be facing forward.

Exercise 6

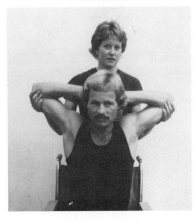

6. With participant sitting and elbows flexed, the assistant places hands on medial side of elbow and pulls elbows back.

Wrist and Finger Exercises (7-17)

Exercise 7

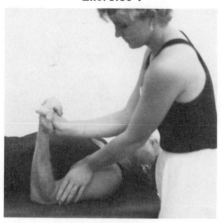

7. With participant supine and elbow flexed, assistant places one hand in palm while the other hand stabilizes upper arm. Assistant pronates and supinates forearm to each end range.

Exercise 8

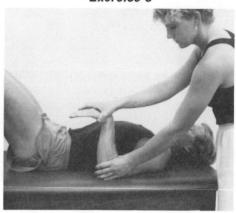

8. With participant supine and elbow flexed, assistant places one hand on dorsum of hand while the other hand stabilizes the elbow. Wrist is flexed to end range.

Exercise 9

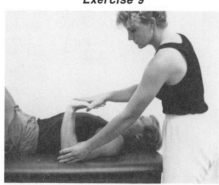

9. With participant supine and elbow flexed, assistant places one hand on palmar surface while the other hand stabilizes elbow. Wrist and fingers are hyperextended to end range.

Exercise 10

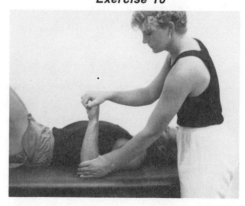

10. With participant supine and elbow flexed, assistant flexes (curls) fingers into a fist.

11. Assistant holds participant's fingers in extension while extending thumb.

Exercise 11

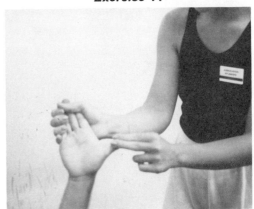

Exercise 12

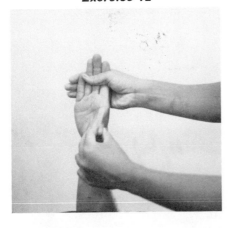

12. Assistant holds participant's fingers in extension while abducting thumb.

Exercise 13

13. With participant supine, assistant places one hand on posterior aspect of thigh while the other hand stabilizes the foot. Assistant flexes hip and knee to end range.

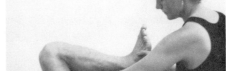

Exercise 14

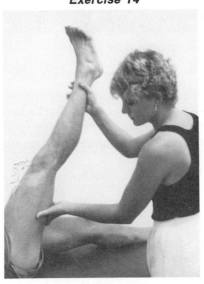

14. With participant supine, assistant places hands on posterior aspect of thigh and lower leg, flexing the hip to end range.

Exercise 15

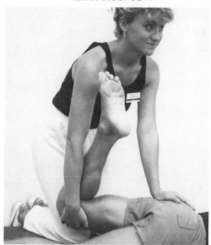

15. With participant prone, assistant places one hand under the anterior aspect of leg, proximal to knee, while stabilizing hip with the other hand. Hip is hyperextended to end range.

Exercise 16

16. With participant side-lying, assistant abducts leg by placing one hand under the medial aspect of the knee joint while the other hand stabilizes the hip.

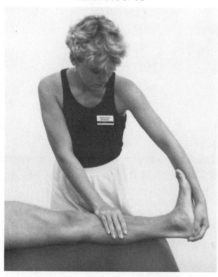

Exercise 17

17. With participant supine, assistant plantar-flexes foot by placing one hand under heel (assistant's forearm rests on plantar surface) while the other hand stabilizes the lower leg.

Wheelchair Stretching Routine Exercises (1-8)

1. Reach one arm across chest. Use other to stretch to end range.

Exercise 1

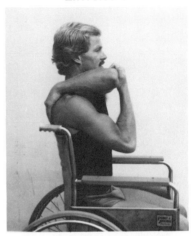

Exercise 2

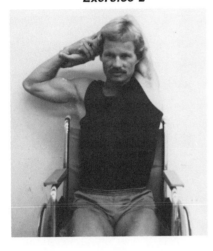

2. Reach arm behind head as if to touch opposite scapula. Use other to stretch arm further.

3. Interlock fingers, keep elbows extended, and flex shoulders, bringing arms above head.

Exercise 3

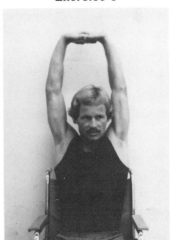

Exercise 4

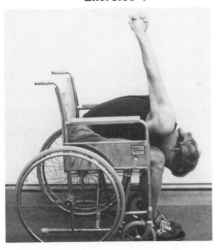

4. Grasp hands behind back and flex forward, attempting to bring hands up as high as possible.

Exercise 5

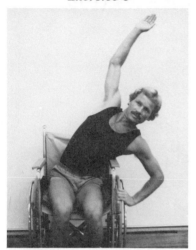

5. Abduct arm (elbow extended) so upper arm is near the ear. Laterally flex trunk. If necessary, hold on to handrim with opposite hand. Repeat to other side.

Exercise 6

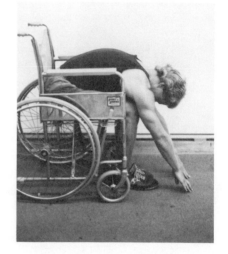

6. Flex forward, reaching hands out in front.

Exercise 7

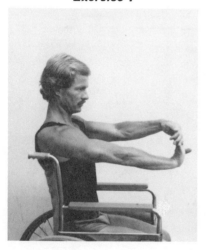

7. Hyperextend wrist and fingers by using other hand to pull back.

Exercise 8

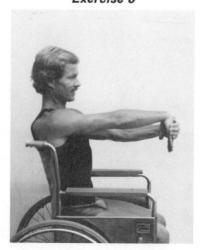

8. Flex wrist by using other hand to pull down.

Study Questions / Learning Activities

1. Outline the optimal conditions for eliciting a stretch.

2. What do you think are the advantages of active stretching over passive techniques (hint: differences in neuromuscular reflex activity, use of voluntary muscle contractions, practicality, liability)?

3. Using a partner, assess active ROM at all major muscle groups. Note any differences between the right and left joints. If any significant bilateral differences are present, question your partner about injuries, habits, or posture that may have contributed to the difference.

4. List contraindications for performing stretching.

5. Describe the techniques used for active stretching, passive stretching, and PNF Hold-Relax.

References

Anderson, B. (1980). *Stretching*. Bolinas, CA: Shelter Publications.

Cornelius, W. L. (1990). Modified PNF stretching: Improvement in hip flexion. *National Strength and Conditioning Association Journal*, 12(4), 44-45.

Hoppenfeld, S. (1976). *Physical examination of the spine and lower extremities*. New York: Appleton-Century-Crofts.

Sapega, A. A., Quenfeld, T. C., Moyer, R. A., & Butler, R.A. (1981). Biophysical factors in range-of-motion exercise. *Physician and sports medicine*, 9(12), 57-65.

Toohey, P., & Larson, C.W. (1977). *Range-of-motion exercise: Key to joint mobility*. Minneapolis: Sister Kennedy Institute.

CHAPTER 8

Assessment and Programming for Cardiovascular Endurance

Assessment of Cardiovascular Endurance

Testing for cardiovascular endurance includes a variety of methods and equipment, reflecting the wide difference in capabilities found among adults with disabilities. This section will provide protocol for submaximal tests in arm crank and wheelchair ergometry, leg cycle ergometry, and jogging.

Arm Crank and Wheelchair Ergometry

Due to lower extremity paralysis found in quadriplegia and paraplegia, arm pedaling or wheelchair pushing have become standard methods for cardiovascular testing. The following is a partial list of ergometric equipment in use today for aerobic testing utilizing the arms (Figoni, 1982):

Wheelchair Treadmills

1. wide (24") electric models, modified to accomodate wheelchair
2. platform with rollers; wheelchair is placed on top

Arm Crank Ergometers

1. friction-braked
   a. Monark rehab trainer or other brand arm crank
   b. leg cycle ergometer interfaced with an arm crank and mounted on table
2. electro-magnetically braked, leg cycle ergometer interfaced with an arm crank and mounted on table

Wheelchair ergometers

1. interfaced with a friction-braked, leg cycle ergometer
2. interfaced with an electro-magnetically braked, leg cycle ergometer

No single test protocol is appropriate to use for all adults with lower extremity paralysis, due to the heterogenous nature of disabilities. Maximal, graded exercise tests have utilized multi-stage, progressive work rates with either continuous or discontinuous protocols. Continuous protocols have used work rate increases every one to six minutes until peak oxygen uptake (VO_2 peak) is achieved. In contrast, discontinuous protocols have typcially used three to six minute bouts with work rate increments separated by one to five minute rest periods. The research literature generally agrees that arm crank and wheelchair ergometry yield a similar VO_2 peak, heart rate, and systolic blood pressure, whether performed as a continuous or discontinuous test. For a more indepth look at different methods of upper extremity testing and training, see the excellent reviews by Franklin (1985), Glaser (1985), and Sawka (1986) in the reference section at the end of this chapter.

The work rate selected for the incremental test has been shown to influence the oxygen uptake achieved (Buchfuhrer et al., 1983; Lasko-McCarthey & Davis, 1991a; Lasko-McCarthey & Davis, 1991b). For persons with quadriplegia due to cervical spinal cord injury, the suggested work rate increment during a continuous test is five watts per minute. For persons with paraplegia, the value can be increased to at least 10 watts per minute. More research is needed to determine suitable work rate increments for other groups with disabilities.

Several factors must be considered when determining heart rate response during maximal graded exeircse testing and subsequent training. Stenberg and associates (1967) demonstrated that the maximal heart rate averages approximately 11 beats per minute lower for arm cycle than for leg cycle exercise. Thus, when using Karvonen's predicted, age-adjusted maximal heart rate (220 - age) for determining work intensity, one must subtract about 10 beats per minute to correct for arm exercise (210 - age).

In spinal cord injuries, especially cervical lesions, paralysis of the trunk and extremities limits significant heart rate increases and venous return of blood. In addition, research has shown that responses of the sympathetic nervous system to exercise become deficient with high thoracic and cervical cord lesions (Knutsson et al., 1973; Nilsson et al., 1975; Wolf & Magora, 1976; Wicks et al., 1983). More specifically, in complete lesions above thoracic nerve root six, inadequate autonomic regulation of the heart restricts the development of exercise tachycardia. Maximal heart rates during exercise are generally restricted to between 100 and 130 beats per minute, even though maximal work rate and muscular effort is present. Thus, heart rate is not a valid physiologic parameter by which to measure the effect of cardiovascular training in persons with high cord lesions. Improvements can be measured via increases in work rate (intensity) and duration of stationary cardiovascular exercise.

Cadence during testing will vary depending upon the equipment used and the ability of the participant. Studies involving arm pedaling have used cadences between 50 and 70 rpm, with 60 rpm being average. In general, lower values have been employed for wheelchair ergometry (e.g., 20 rpm).

Precautions During Testing

1. Use a fan to facilitate the dissipation of body heat generated during aerobic exercise. Perspiring does not occur below the level of the spinal cord lesion in persons with complete injuries. Persons with cervical spinal cord injury are especially prone to overheating. Excessive heat is a major contributor of fatigue in persons with multiple sclerosis.
2. Persons with spinal cord injury should empty the bladder prior to exercise to minimize the effects on circulation of hyperactive distension reflexes or autonomic dysreflexia (Knutsson et al., 1973).
3. When testing untrained or elderly individuals, closely monitor the cardiovascular responses until it is determined that normal responses are present (heart rate, heart rhythm, and blood pressure). Continue to periodically check these variables.
4. If a feeling of faintness occurs due to orthostatic reactions (e.g., venous pooling, sluggish blood pressure), place individual in a horizontal position or sit with head below waist. The level of injury is not entirely accurate in determining orthostatic reactions.

Protocol for Submaximal Arm Ergometry Test
(for use with Monark Rehab Trainer or other arm crank ergometer)

1. The evaluation form used in conjunction with this test is provided in the next section (see "Arm and Leg Cycle Ergometers - Submaximal Exercise Test").
2. Adjust the height of the arm crank so that the fulcrum is at shoulder level.
3. Take a resting heart rate and blood pressure.
4. If necessary, bind the participant's hands to the pedals with elastic bandage.
5. Lock brakes on the wheelchair to prevent excessive movement.
6. Use a metronome to establish the cadence. Have participant begin pedaling and start the stopwatch.

    Persons with quadriplegia: 50-65 rpm
    Persons with paraplegia: 60-70 rpm

    A pace of 65 rpm is generally considered to be the most mechanically efficient, although efficiency will depend upon the work rate. Efficiency is greater at higher work rates when the cadence is higher. The converse is true for lower work rates.

    Cadence should stay constant throughout test.
7. Work stages are two minutes in duration.
8. Begin with zero load as a warm up for two minutes.

9. The work rate increment after warm up will vary according to individual capabilities and training level. See the last section of this chapter for computing work rates based on kiloponds, cadence, and wheel circumference. Average work rate increments are suggested below:

    Persons with quadriplegia pedaling at 50 rpm:

    1/4 kp per stage (37.5 kpm/min or 6 watts).

    Persons with paraplegia pedaling at 60 rpm:

    1/4 - 1/2 kp per stage (45 - 90 kpm or 7.4 to 14.7 watts, respectively)

10. Following each stage, provide a one minute rest period when heart rate and blood pressure are taken. Then resume the test by having participant begin pedaling; increase work rate by designated increment once cadence is achieved.

11. Do not test individuals with resting blood pressure exceeding 140/90 without prior medical approval. The normal responses of blood pressure to exercise are the following: Systolic - progressive increase with incremental work rates. Diastolic - no change or slight decrease (10 mm Hg during progressive workloads).

12. For individuals with lesions above thoracic nerve root six, the heart rate response will not correlate well with effort; thus, continue to test until volitional fatigue is reached.

13. If the participant experiences pain or pressure in the chest, pain radiating into the left arm and/or jaw, nausea, faintness, or troublesome shortness of breath, the test must be discontinued. See Contraindications for Exercise Testing and Indications for Terminating an Exercise Test in Chapter 15. Submaximal tests with persons over 40 years of age should be discontinued if the heart rate exceeds 140 beats per minute.

14. For persons under 40 years of age and without any cardiovascular restrictions, continue to test until a heart rate is achieved that represents 70-80% of the predicted, age adjusted, maximal heart rate for arm work (using Karvonen's formula). The work rate achieved at this stage will serve as the work rate used during training.

15. After the cessation of the test, the participant should warm down for several minutes at zero load. Stay with participant and monitor heart rate and blood pressure every couple of minutes until values have returned to resting levels.

16. At the end of the program, use the identical protocol to post-test the participant. Compare the heart rate achieved at each stage to pretest values. If a training effect has occurred, the heart rates should be lower in post-test when compared to the pretest. This result indicates that the delivery and utilization of oxygen has become more efficient and hence a lower heart rate to accomplish the same submaximal task.

17. If heart rate is not a valid parameter for measuring improvement in the subject (i.e., high thoracic or cervical spinal cord injury), then conduct the post-test identical to the pretest but continue to test the subject at higher work rates until volitional fatigue is attained. If a training effect has occurred over the course of the program, then accumulated work will be higher in the post-test than pretest (total sum of work performed during the test - add up kpm/min).

Testing Protocol for Submaximal Leg Cycle Ergometry (use with Monark, Bodyguard, or other friction-braked cycle)

1. Use the same evaluation form as for arm crank ergometry.
2. The seat height should be adjusted so when the front part of the foot is on the pedal, there is approximately 15 degrees of flexion in the knee. This is the most effective position during heavy work.
3. Take a resting heart rate and blood pressure. Do not test a participant with a blood pressure greater than 140/90 without medical consultation.
4. With the subject seat on the bicycle, but without touching the pedals, set the mark on the pendulum to "0" on the scale.
5. Use a metronome to establish the one of the suggested cadences below:
    - 50 rpm   person who is untrained, elderly, or disabled
    - 60-70 rpm   person who is trained
6. Begin the test with the brake belt slack. When the correct cadence is achieved, set the desired work rate and start the stopwatch. Suggested incremental work rates:
    - Person who is untrained, elderly, or disabled pedaling at 50 rpm:
        - 1/2 kp per stage (150 kpm/min or 24.4 watts).
    - Person who is trained pedaling at 60 rpm:
        - 1 kp per stage (360 kpm/min or 58.8 watts).
7. Three minute work stages should be used.
8. Increase the work rate by the designated increment for each stage.
9. Take heart rate and blood pressure at the end of each stage (last 15 seconds) while the subject continues to pedal.
10. For persons under 40 years of age and without any cardiovascular restrictions, continue to test until a heart rate is achieved that represents 70-80% of the predicted, age-adjusted, maximal heart rate for leg work (using Karvonen's formula). The work rate achieved at this stage will serve as the work rate used during training. Discontinue the test if the heart rate rises above 140 beats per minute for elderly participants.
11. Do not test individuals with resting blood pressure exceeding 140/90 without prior medical approval. The normal responses of blood pressure to exercise are the following: Systolic - progressive increase with incremental work rates. Diastolic - no change or slight decrease (10 mm Hg during progressive workloads).
12. If the participant experiences pain or pressure in the chest, pain radiating into the left arm and/or jaw, nausea, faintness, or troublesome shortness of breath, the test must be discontinued. See Contraindications for Exercise Testing and Indications for Terminating an Exercise Test in Chapter 15.
13. After the cessation of the test, the participant should warm down for several minutes at zero load. Stay with participant and monitor heart rate and blood pressure every couple of minutes until values have returned to resting levels.
14. At the end of the program, use the identical protocol to post-test the participant. Compare the heart rate achieved at each stage to pretest values. If a training effect has occurred, the heart rates should be lower in post-test when compared to the pretest. This result indicates that the delivery and utlization of oxygen has become more efficient and hence a lower heart rate to accomplish the same submaximal task.

Arm and Leg Cycle Ergometers
Submaximal Exercise Test

NAME_____ DATE_____ AGE_____ SEX_____

HEIGHT_____in. WEIGHT_____lb. PREDICTED MAXIMUM HEART RATE_____bpm

#1 PRE-SEMESTER WORK TEST: DATE OF TEST_____ TIME OF DAY_____

RESTING HR_____bpm RESTING BP (mm Hg) #1_____ #2_____ #3_____ TARGET HR_____bpm

Time (min)	Load (kp)	Rate (rpm)	Work Rate (kpm/min)	Heart Rate (bpm)	Blood Pressure (mm Hg)	Mets	Comments/Symptons
0-2	Rec.						
4-5	Rec.						

#2 MID-SEMESTER WORK TEST: DATE OF TEST_____ TIME OF DAY_____

RESTING HR_____bpm RESTING BP (mm Hg) #1_____ #2_____ #3_____ TARGET HR_____bpm

Time (min)	Load (kp)	Rate (rpm)	Work Rate (kpm/min)	Heart Rate (bpm)	Blood Pressure (mm Hg)	Mets	Comments/Symptons
0-2	Rec.						
4-5	Rec.						

#3 POST-SEMESTER WORK TEST: DATE OF TEST_____ TIME OF DAY_____

RESTING HR_____bpm RESTING BP (mm Hg) #1_____ #2_____ #3_____ TARGET HR_____bpm

Time (min)	Load (kp)	Rate (rpm)	Work Rate (kpm/min)	Heart Rate (bpm)	Blood Pressure (mm Hg)	Mets	Comments/Symptons
0-2	Rec.						
4-5	Rec.						

Assessment of Cardiovascular Endurance in Ambulatory Persons

There are several simple methods to assess cardiovascular endurance in ambulatory persons. The two most common methods are the 12 minute Run-Walk and the Step Test.

12 Minute Run-Walk

The goal of this test is to have the participant cover as much distance as possible in 12 minutes. It is best to perform the test on track for ease of calculations. It is useful to place cones every 100 yards to facilitate measurement of distance. For norms, see Cooper (1977) in the reference section at the end of this chapter. This test can be used to compare pre-training and post-training levels of aerobic fitness.

Step Test

Another practical test that requires very little equipment is the Step Test. This test, along with the bicycle ergometer, is excellent for assessing visually impaired students. This test is also appropriate for all ages and both sexes. Because the test lasts only three minutes, only extremely unfit individuals would find this test too vigorous. Obviously, this test should only be performed if the participant has been given a medical clearance by a physician.

The protocol of the test involves stepping up and down on a 12-inch high bench for three minutes at a pace of 24 steps per minute. After three minutes, immediately take the pulse. For further clarification of the test and listing of norms, see Kasch and Boyer (1968) in the reference section at the end of this chapter.

Programming for Cardiovascular Endurance

Part of the disuse syndrome that occurs when an individual is immobilized is the loss of cardiovascular endurance. This reduction in aerobic capacity has many health implications in regards to obesity and heart disease. Regular, moderate physical activity may aid efforts to control cigarette smoking, hypertension, lipid abnormalities, diabetes, obesity, and emotional stress (American Heart Association, 1981). The following section provides some guidelines for instituting a cardiovascular training program for non-ambulatory participants.

Arm Crank Ergometry

Duration of Exercise

Studies involving arm pedaling have primarily used interval training for improving fitness parameters of those with lower extremity disabilities. Significant improvements in physiologic responses have occurred using three, four-minute work bouts separated by two-minute rest intervals (Glasser et al., 1981; Glaser, 1985). Pollock and associates (1974) alternated one minute bouts of high and low work rates, progressing to 30 minutes of continuous high work rate by the 19th week of training for persons with paraplegia. See Table 8-1 for suggested interval training programs for persons with quadriplegia and paraplegia.

Frequency of Exercise

Researchers generally agree that frequency of training should occur between three to five times per week.

Intensity of Exercise - Target Heart Rate

The purpose of the target heart rate (THR) is to establish the intensity of exercise necessary to produce a training effect on the cardiovascular system. Several factors must be considered when determining THR for arm crank ergometry. The maximal heart rate averages about 10 beats lower for arm than for leg work. Thus, when using Karvonen's predicted, age-adjusted maximal heart rate (220 - age) for determining work intensity, subtract 10 beats to correct for arm exercise (i.e., 210 - age). Resting heart rates can be obtained by taking a 60 second count prior to the exercise bout.

Karvonen's Formula

Example:

210		210
- ___	Subtract age	- 20
___	Predicted, age-adjusted maximum	190
- ___	Subtract resting heart rate	- 70
___	Heart rate reserve	120
x ___	Multiply by exercise intensity of 60-80%	x .70
		84
+ ___	Add resting heart rate back in	+ 70
___	**Target heart rate (beats/min)**	**154**

The percentage entered into the formula for the intensity depends on how much training one has had in the past. The following percentages are recommended:

Over 30 years of age	beginning	60-70%
College age	beginning	70-80%
Trained	less than two years	75-85%
Trained	more than two years	85-95%

Due to disturbances in the sympathetic nervous system and partial paralysis of the arm and shoulder musculature, persons with spinal cord lesions above thoracic nerve root six cannot use Karvonen's formula because of deficient exercise tachycardia. The heart rate reaches a ceiling between approximately 100-130 beats/minute. Therefore, the individual at this type of disability should attempt to achieve his/her ceiling heart rate during training bouts.

Training Cadence (revolutions per minute)

Persons with quadriplegia: 50-65 rpm
Persons with paraplegia: 60-70 rpm

Recording on the Exercise Program Card

Designate on the program card which mode of exercise is being used (arm or leg cycling), the cadence, and target heart rate. Allow space for recording the work rate (or kiloponds) and duration of **each** work bout. Also record on a daily basis the resting and exercising heart rates and blood pressures. See Chapter 1 (page 9) for a sample exercise program card with arm ergometry.

Note
The same precautions that apply to arm crank testing should be followed for arm crank training.

Table 8-1. *Interval Training for Adults with Quadriplegia and Paraplegia*

Level of Lesion	Pace	Duration	Intensity	Frequenty
C-4 to C-8	50-65 rpm	30 sec. work, 30 sec. rest until fatigue or 3 bouts: 2-4 min. each, 2-3 min. rest	Ceiling HR	3-5 x/week
T-1 to T-6	60-70 rpm	3 bouts: 4 min. each, 2 min. rest or 1 min. high load, 1 min. low load for 10-30 min.	same	same
T-7 and below	same	same	70-80% of max (Karvonen's formula)	same

Leg Cycle Ergometry

The guidelines for leg cycle ergometry are very similar to those presented for arm crank ergometry. Precautions and contraindications for that were presented for testing should be reviewed.

Duration

Interval training may be used for those initially beginning a cycling program. The work and rest periods will vary depending upon the individual. Three bouts are recommended with approximately two minutes of rest between each. The duration of each bout will depend upon the age, training level, and disability of the participant. If a continuous training bout is used, 15 to 60 minutes is suggested.

Intensity

Use Karvonen's formula for determining the THR. A modified version of this formula was presented earlier. The same formula should be used but with the following change:

$$\frac{\begin{array}{r} 220 \\ -\underline{\hspace{1cm}} \text{ (age)} \end{array}}{\underline{\hspace{1cm}} \text{ (age-adjusted, predicted maximum HR)}}$$

After this computation, the remainder of the formula can be used. The same guidelines for selection of intensity that were used for arm crank ergometry may be applied to leg work.

Frequency

Three to five days a week are recommended.

How to Take Pulse

1. Take pulse at the thumb side of the wrist on the palm or inner side of the forearm, as shown in Figure 8-1. Place your fingers at the area marked "X" and you will feel a throb there. Do not use your thumb because it has it's own pulse.
2. Look at the second hand of a clock and count how many beats you feel in 10 seconds. Multiply this number by six to obtain the pulse for one minute. If the pulse is weak and irregular, count for a full minute.
3. If the pulse is difficult to feel or cannot be found at the wrist, use the temple or under the jaw at the carotid artery as shown in the following illustration.

Locations for Taking Pulse

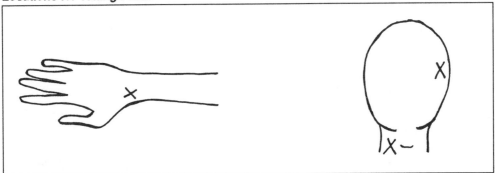

Calculating Work Rate for Arm and Leg Cycle Ergometers (Monark, Bodyguard, and other friction-braked ergometers)

The circumference of the ergometer wheel typically equals 6 meters on leg cycles and 3 meters on arm cycles. If the cadence is 50 rpm, the distance covered would be 300 and 150 meters per minute, respectively.

The wheel is mechanically braked by a belt strapped around the rim. This belt is adjusted by a hand-turned wheel, providing resistance that is measured in kiloponds. A kilopond is the force acting upon the mass of one kilogram at normal acceleration of gravity.

Computation for Work Rate

kp * m/min = kpm/min

Where

kp = number of kiloponds set by adjustment of belt tension

m/min = distance pedaled in meters per minute (multiply circumference of wheel by rpm)

A kilopond meter (kpm) is defined as the work necessary to lift a one kilogram mass one meter against normal gravitational force. Expressed per minute, the work rate is written as kpm/min. A watt is a unit of power equal to 6.12 kpm/min.

Study Questions / Learning Activities

1. List the modes of exercise available for testing persons with lower extremity paralysis.

2. List the precautions to follow during testing of persons with spinal cord injury.

3. Use Karvonen's Formula to compute your target heart rate.

4. Explain why persons with high thoracic and cervical spinal cord lesions can not use Karvonen's Formula for determining target heart rate.

5. Administer a submaximal, incremental exercise test to a partner, using an arm crank ergometer. If a device is not available, place a leg cycle ergometer on a table.

6. Prescribe a training program based on your test results.

7. Compute work rates (kpm/min and watts) for the following data:

    1 kilopond at 300 m/min
    2 kiloponds at 600 m/min
    .5 kilopond at 180 m/min

References

AAHPERD health-related fitness test. AAHPERD Publications, 1900 Association Drive, Reston, VA, 22091.

American College of Sportsmedicine (1983). *Reference guide for workshop/ certification programs in preventive/rehabilitative exercise.*

American College of Sports Medicine (1986, 3rd ed.). *Guidelines for exercise testing and prescription.* Philadelphia: Lea and Febiger, p. 7.

American Heart Association. Subcommittee on Exercise/Cardiac Rehabilitation (1981). Statement on exercise. *Circulation, 64,* 1302A.

Buchfuhrer, M. J., Hansen, J. E., Robinson, T. E., Sue, Y. D., Wasserman, K., & Whipp, B. J. Optimizing the exercise protocol for cardiopulmonary assessment. *Journal of Applied Physiology, 55,* 558-564.

Chawla, J. C., Bar, D., Creber, I., Price, J., & Andrew, B. (1980). Techniques for improving the strength and fitness of spinal cord injured patients. *Paraplegia, 17,* 185-190.

Davis, G. M., Shephard, R. J., & Jackson, R. W. (1981). Cardio-respiratory fitness and muscular strength in the lower-limb disabled. *Canadian Journal of Applied Sport Sciences, 6*(4), 159-165.

Dearwater, S.P., LaPorte, R.E., Robertson, R. J., Brenes, G., Adams, L.L., & Becker, D. (1986). Activity in the spinal cord-injured patient: an epidemiologic analysis of metabolic parameters. *Medicine and Science in Sports and Exercise, 18,* 541-544.

Dreisinger, T. E., Whiting, R. V., & Hayden, C. R. (1982). Wheelchair exercise testing: comparison of continuous and discontinuous tests. *Medicine and Science in Sports and Exercise, 14*(2), 168.

Figoni, S. F. (1984). Spinal cord injury and maximal aerobic power. *American Corrective Therapy Journal, 38,* 44-50.

Fox, S. M., Naughton, S. P., & Haskell, W .L. (1971). Physical activity and the prevention of coronary heart disease. *Annuals of Clinical Research, 3,* 404.

Franklin, B. (1985). Exercise testing, training and arm ergometry. *Sports Medicine, 2,* 100-119.

Gass, G. C., & Camp, E. M. (1979). Physiological characteristics of trained Australian paraplegic and tetraplegic subjects. *Medicine and Science in Sports and Exercise, 11,* 256-259.

Glaser, R. M. (1985). Exercise and locomotion for the spinal cord injured. In: *Exercise and Sport Sciences Reviews,* R. L. Terjung (Ed.). New York: Macmillan, pp. 263-303.

Golding, L. A., Horvat, M. A., Beutel-Horvat, T., & McConnell, T. J. (1986). A graded exercise test protocol for spinal cord injured individuals. *Journal of Cardiopulmonary Rehabilitation, 6,* 362-367.

Haskins, M. (1972). *Evaluation in physical education.* Dubuque: W. C. Brown.

Hooker, S. P., & Wells, C. L. (1989). Effects of low- and moderate-intensity training in spinal cord-injured persons. *Medicine and Science in Sports and Exercise, 21,* 18-22.

Knutson, E., Lewnhaupt-Olsen, E., & Thorsen, M. (1973). Physical capacity and physical conditioning in paraplegic patients. *Paraplegia, 11,* 205-216.

Lasko-McCarthey, P., & Davis, J.A. (1991a). Protocol dependency of $\dot{V}O_2$ max during arm cycle ergometry in males with quadriplegia. *Medicine and Science in Sports and Exercise, 23*(9), 1097-1101.

Lasko-McCarthey, P., & Davis, J.A. (1991b). Effect of work rate increment on peak oxygen uptake during wheelchair ergometry in men with quadriplegia. *European Journal of Applied Physiology, 63,* 349-353.

Nilsson, S., Staff, P. H., & Pruett, E. D. R. (1975). Physical work capacity and the effect of training on subjects with long-standing paraplegia. *Scandinavian Journal of Rehabilitative Medicine, 7,* 51-56.

Pollock, M. L., Miller, H. S., Linnerud, A. C., Laughridge, E., Coleman, E., & Alexander, E. (1974). Arm pedaling as an endurance training regimen for the disabled. *Archives of Physical Medicine Rehabilitation, 55,* 252-261.

Sawka, M. (1986). Physiology of upper body exercise. In: *Exercise and sport sciences reviews,* R. L. Terjung (Ed.). New York: Macmillan, pp. 175-211.

Wicks, J. R., Oldridge, N. B., Cameron, B. J., & Jones, N. L. (1983). Arm cranking and wheelchair ergometry in elite spinal cord-injured athletes. *Medicine and Science in Sports and Exercise, 15,* 224-231.

Assessment and Programming for Gait

Assessment of Gait

The assessment of gait may range from simple clinical observations to complex laboratory tests with video tape, digitization, force plate switches, and electromyography. This chapter will focus on utilizing clinical observations and a simple quantitative method for assessing gait. For safety and liability purposes, the adapted physical educator should obtain medical clearance prior to assessing the gait pattern and implementing an exercise program. This recommendation is strongly urged because if the participant has not stood or walked for an extended period of time, bones may be osteoporotic, strength may be diminished, and balance may be impaired.

The Step Cycle of Normal Gait

Normal gait is typically evaluated by examining the gait or step cycle. The step cycle is defined as the period from heelstrike to heelstrike of the same foot. There are two phases in the step cycle (see Figure 9-1):

Stance phase (comprises 60% of step cycle)
- Period of partial or full weight bearing.
- Begins with heelstrike and ends when same foot is plantarflexed in toe-off and weight is shifted to other extremity.
- Divided into three stages known as heelstrike, midstance (weight shifted from heel to ball of foot), and toe-off.

Swing Phase (comprises 40% of step cycle)
- Begins as weight is shifted off extremity with accompanying hip and knee flexion. Ends when knee is in full extension prior to heelstrike.
- Divided into three stages known as acceleration, midswing, and deceleration.

One Step Cycle of Normal Gait

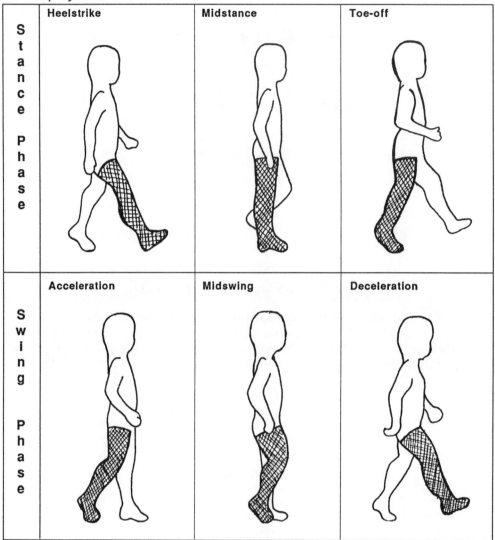

Components of Normal Gait (Daniels & Worthingham, 1972; Hoppenfeld, 1976)

1. Head erect.
2. Shoulders level.
3. Trunk vertical.
4. Base of support: 2 to 4 inches from heel to heel.
5. Arms swing reciprocally and with equal amplitude.
6. Steps are the same length.
7. Vertical oscillations of the center of gravity (COG) are about 2 inches and even in tempo.

8. Knee flexes in stance (except at heelstrike) to prevent excessive vertical rise in the COG.
9. Pelvis slightly rotates in the transverse plane (4 degrees).
10. Pelvis tilts in the frontal plane (5 degrees downward).
11. Pelvis laterally tilts toward the supporting leg.
12. Pelvis and trunk shift laterally approximately 1 inch toward the supporting leg to center the body weight over the hip.
13. During swing, the pelvis rotates 40 degrees forward and the opposite hip acts a fulcrum for rotation.
14. Average walking speed: 3 feet/second or 2-2.5 mph.
15. Average cadence: 90-120 steps/minute.
16. Average step length: 15 inches.

Clinical Observation of Gait

1. If possible, have the participant walk barefoot in short pants or swimsuit.
2. If possible, observe the participant walking both with and without supportive devices and/or ambulation aids.
3. Ask the participant to walk about 25 feet away from the examiner. If possible, the participant should make several excursions to allow observations from anterior, posterior, and lateral views, and to determine any consistent patterns.
4. If possible, observe the participant walking at several speeds, ascending/descending stairs, and sitting/rising.
5. Note any dominant positions/posture of the arms, trunk, and legs.
6. Observe the stance phase first. Many problems become distinct during this phase because it accounts for 60% of the step cycle and the affected extremity must assume full weight bearing during this period.
7. Observe body segments separately (i.e., foot, knee, hip, trunk, and arms) in anterior, posterior, and lateral views.
8. Listen as well as look for disorders. Certain gait abnormalities will result in an uneven step tempo, slapping or scraping sounds.

Quantitative Gait Evaluation (see "Gait Analysis" form)

A simple method was developed by Robinson and Smidt (1981) which calculates the following temporal and distance factors of gait: velocity, cadence, stride length, and step length. This quantitative form of evaluation allows one to determine improvements which may not be readily observable to the eye. The method requires very little equipment (homemade grid floor pattern, stopwatch, tape measure, and portable tape recorder) and a minimum of space and time. More specific details of the method can be found in the publication by Robinson and Smidt entitled, "Quantitative Gait Evaluation in the Clinic," *Physical Therapy*, March, 1981 (volume 61, number 3).

Abnormal Gait Patterns (Dunn, 1982)

Gait Pattern	Characteristics
Antalgic	• Pain on weightbearing • Quick stance on affected lower extremity (LE) • Short stride (swing) • Less flexion of affected LE

Ataxic
   cerebellar
 	
   spinal
	
	• Wide-based, staggering gait
	• Loss of stability with eyes open or closed
	• Unilateral lesions result in sway toward side of lesion
	• May have foot stamping
	
	• Loss of position sense with eyes closed (involvement of proprioceptive pathways)
	• May evidence foot foot slap

Festinating	• Short, accelerating shuffling steps
Dystrophic	• Wide-based waddling gait with lateral lurch and trunk hyperextended.
Spastic/Scissors	• Excessive hip flexion, internal rotation, and adduction • Knee flexion or extension • Ankles may be plantarflexed • Knees cross in front of one another during gait due to spasticity • Toes may drag
Steppage/Dropfoot	• Excess hip and knee flexion during swing due to foot drop (flaccid dorsiflexors) • Instead of heelstrike the foot strike is plantigrade (flat foot landing)
Trendelenburg	• Gluteus medius lurch • Exaggerated drop of the pelvis toward unaffected side during stance phase of the affected extremity
Circumducted	• During swing, the hip is circumducted so the lower leg and foot clear the ground • May also involve tilting the pelvis upward

GAIT ANALYSIS

Name ———————————————————— Date————————

Disability ——————————————————————————

Ambulatory Aids———————————————————————

GAIT PATTERN	RIGHT	LEFT
1. Antalgic		
2. Ataxic		
3. Festinating		
4. Dystrophic/Waddling		
5. Spastic/Scissors		
6. Steppage		
7. Trendelenburg		
8. Circumducted		
9. Foot		
10. Hip/Knee		
11. Trunk/Arms		
12. Other		

TEMPORAL AND DISTANCE FACTORS

1. Average Velocity   = ——————in ——————sec

                              = ——————in/sec

2. Average Cadence (90-120) = ——————steps/sec * 60

                              = ——————steps/min

3. Average Stride Length   = R ——————in

4. Average Step Length   = R ——————in

                                L ——————in

Programming for Gait Training

Role of the Adapted Physical Educator in Gait Training (Mason & Dando, 1979)

Development of Strength and Endurance in Muscles Utilized in Walking

This development includes muscles of the lower extremities, particularly the flexors and extensors of the hip, knee, and ankle. Strengthening muscles of the trunk aids further stability during walking. Whenever possible, strength should be developed in whole patterns of movement (i.e., multi-joint movement) rather than single joint movement. This technique will allow more transfer of strength and coordination.

Development of Even Length and Timing of Steps

The length of the step on the affected extremity will be shortened. The participant should be encouraged to take larger steps on the affected side. A metronome may be utilized to aid with tempo of steps.

Instruction in Proper Placement of Feet, Legs, Trunk, and Arms to Facilitate Stability and Coordination

Consistent cues and constant feedback should be provided to the participant by the assistant. This practice requires careful observation by the assistant. Skill feedback is usually provided in the following areas:

1. heel-strike (heel-to-toe progression of the foot).
2. direction of forefoot (should point slightly out from line of travel).
3. degree of flexion or hyperextension in the knee.
4. lateral tilt of the pelvis.
5. anterior tilt of the pelvis.
6. erect trunk and head
7. relaxed, reciprocal movement of the arms.

Development of Dynamic Balance and Transfer of Weight

See "Exercises for Developing Static and Dynamic Balance" provided in Chapter 10 starting on page 138.

Development of Flexibility

Contractures and spasticity may interfere with standing and the gait pattern. See Chapter 7 for specific stretching techniques.

Progression in Gait Training

1. Standing Frame
2. Kinetron
3. Parallel Bars

4. Walker
5. Crutch
6. Cane

Kinetron Progression

Purpose - to develop

1. weight-bearing strength and endurance.
2. range of motion in the hip, knee, and ankle.
3. power (quickness) in lower extremity extension and flexion;
   i.e., development of necessary forces quickly enough for efficient ambulation.
4. coordination of weight transfer (reciprocate bilaterally).

Positioning

1. adjust the length of kinetron arm so the foot pedals are at a comfortable distance from the seat.
2. height of the actuator sets the degree of hip and knee flexion.
3. height of seat determines the degree of hip and knee extension desired in the pattern of movement and the height of the arm rest.
4. speed selector dials establishes the speed of movement on left and right sides.

Testing

1. Warm-up: 10 submaximal efforts
2. Have participant perform a maximal thrust (hip and knee extension) on both affected and unaffected extremities at a selected speed. The highest reading on the gauge for the unaffected leg then becomes the goal for the affected leg.

Progression

1. Retrain the ability to reciprocate bilaterally.
2. Develop measured levels of weight-bearing. Achieve pressure gauge reading of 100-150 psi at all speeds. Begin at speeds of 1, 2, or 3 and progress to higher speeds. If necessary, the affected side may work at a slower speed to achieve 100-150 psi while the unaffected side continues to work submaximally at 3. When increasing the speed beyond 3, work both sides together. For strength, use a speed setting of 4. For functional strength, use a speed setting of 5.
3. If necessary, use weights on rear tube of unaffected side to allow for passive extension of affected leg.

4. Begin with 3 sets of 10 repetitions (strength) and progress to continuous 1-2 minute intervals (endurance).
5. To achieve a more vertical position:
   - raise seat height
   - shorten arm length
   - bring seat back forward
6. Have the individual strive to raise the foot (during knee and hip flexion) ahead of the rising footplate.

Gait Training Using Parallel Bars

Gait training using parallel bars can be found under "Exercises for Developing Static and Dynamic Balance" in Chapter 10 on page 138.

Gait Training With Crutches and Canes

There are approximately nine different types of crutch gaits. Selection depends upon the participant's ability to take steps with either or both of the lower extremities (Sorenson & Ulrich, 1977).

Four-Point Alternate Gait

1. right crutch
2. left foot
3. left crutch
4. right foot

Two-Point Alternate Gait

1. right crutch and left foot (simultaneously)
2. left crutch and right foot (simultaneously)

Three-Point Gait

1. both crutches and the weak extremity
2. strong lower extremity

Tripod Alternating Gait

1. right crutch
2. left crutch
3. drag body

Tripod Simultaneous Gait

1. both crutches (simultaneously)
2. drag body, both legs (simultaneously)

Swing-to-Gait

1. both crutches (simultaneously)
2. lift body and swing legs (simultaneously) to crutches

Swing-Through Gait

1. both crutches, simultaneously
2. lift both legs and swing beyond crutches (simultaneously)

Rocking Chair Gait

1. both crutches
2. one foot, alternating with
3. the other foot

Two Point Amputation Gait

1. right foot and right crutch (simultaneously)
2. left foot and left crutch (simultaneously)

Crutch Activities (Mason & Dando, 1978)

1. walking backward and sideward.
2. turning around.
3. opening and closing doors.
4. sitting down and standing up.
5. ascending and descending ramps, stairs, and curbs.
6. getting to and from floor from a standing position.
7. falling safely.
8. going over obstacles.
9. picking up objects from the floor.
10. carrying objects.

Ascending and Descending Stairs

When Ascending Stairs

1. step up with the stronger leg
2. bring up ambulation aid (if being used)
3. bring up the weaker leg

When Descending Stairs:

1. bring down ambulation aid (if being used)
2. step down with weaker leg
3. bring down the stronger leg

Additional Ambulation Exercises (De Anza College, CA)

1. forward walking
2. backward walking
3. side walking
4. cross-over sideways - front and back
5. knee bends
6. high knee walking
7. bent knee walking
8. step over obstacles
9. treadmill - 1 mph, 3% grade
10. metronome walking
11. obstacle course
12. bicycle (stationary and three wheel)

Additional Teaching Tips

1. If a participant has difficulty with coordinating a reciprocal arm swing, have him/her hold a cane in each hand. An assistant should stand behind the participant, grasp the canes, and manually assist the participant to achieve the proper coordination during walking.
2. A walking belt should be wore by the participant during gait training. This belt provides the assistant with a grip to aid the participant in stability.
3. If a participant collapses during gait training, the assistant should not attempt to hold the person up but break the fall by slowly lowering him/her to the ground with an eccentric contraction of the legs. This maneuver prevents injury to the assistant's back.
4. Sensory loss (proprioception) in the upper and lower extremities may affect balance and confidence during gait training. Use a mirror whenever possible and provide feedback regarding body positions.
5. If the participant is using only one cane or crutch, make sure it is placed in the hand opposite the extremity.
6. Adjust the height of parallel bars, canes, or crutches to allow for 15-30 degrees of flexion at the elbow.

Study Questions / Learning Activities

1. Identify and define the two phases of the step cycle.

2. List 10 components of normal gait.

3. Using a partner, follow the procedures for clinical observation of gait. Note any deviations from a normal pattern.

4. Describe the spastic, steppage, and circumducted gait patterns. Utilize Chapter 13 to determine which disabilities may result in these gait patterns.

5. Describe the five roles of the adapted physical educator in regards to gait training.

6. Have a partner demonstrate a crutch gait pattern - identify which pattern is being performed.

References

Daniels, L., & Worthingham, C. (1972). *Muscle testing*. Philadelphia: W. B. Saunders.

De Anza College (1984). *Adapted physical education manual*. Cupertino, CA.

Hoppenfeld, S. (1976). *Physical examination of the spine and extremities*. New York: Appleton-Century-Crofts.

Mason, E., & Dando, H. (1975). *Corrective therapy and adapted physical education*. Chillicothe, Ohio: American Corrective Therapy Association.

Sorenson, L., & Ulrich, P.G. (1977, 2nd ed.). *Ambulation guide for nurses*. Minneapolis: Sister Kennedy Institute.

CHAPTER 10

Assessment and Programming for Perceptual-Motor Skills

Definition of the Perceptual-Motor Process

The perceptual-motor process can be viewed as a continuous cycle of the following events:

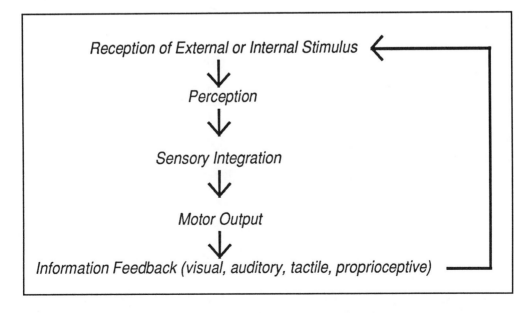

Reception of External or Internal Stimulus

↓

Perception

↓

Sensory Integration

↓

Motor Output

↓

Information Feedback (visual, auditory, tactile, proprioceptive)

According to Harris (1983), the term perception refers to " ... the detection, recognition, discrimination, and interpretation of simple stimuli received through the individual sense modalities." Four regions of the brain which are responsible for perception are: (1) cerebral cortex, (2) thalamus, (3) hypothalamus, and (4) cerebellum (Sherrill, 1986).

The following disabilities are typically associated with perceptual-motor deficiencies: learning disabilities, mental retardation, acquired brain injury, spinal bifida, cerebral palsy, multiply sclerosis, ataxia, stroke, and aphasia. The natural course of aging can diminish perceptual-motor skills due to degeneration of the central and peripheral nervous systems. Perceptual-motor impairments are also associated with the following behavioral traits (Lerch et al., 1974): hyperactivity, emotional lability, short attention span, distractibility, and impulsivity.

Perceptual-motor tests which are standardized and norm-referenced for the adult do not exist. Therefore, the adapted physical educator at the post-secondary level must design a criterion-referenced test or survey. The instructor can borrow items from formal perceptual-motor tests for children. Criterion-referenced test items specify a skill (e.g., static balance on one foot), the test conditions (e.g., opposite knee flexed 90 degrees, hands on hips, eyes open), and the criterion for passing (e.g., 10 seconds without falling). The survey should be comprehensive in scope to accomodate the heterogeneous nature of persons with disabilities. The most frequently assessed areas in perceptual-motor functioning are listed below.

Most Frequently Assessed Areas in Perceptual-Motor Functioning

Gross Motor
Balance
   Static
   Dynamic
Intersensory Coordination
   Eye-Hand
   Eye-Foot
Kinesthesis
   Body Awareness
   Laterality (awareness of right and left)
   Bilateral Coordination or Integration
Motor planning (praxia)

Fine Motor
Intersensory Coordination
   Eye-Hand (e.g., copying shapes, buttoning, cutting)
   Kinesthesis (e.g., finger opposition)

Visual Perception
Spatial Awareness/Orientation
Figure-Ground
Memory
Discrimination
Ocular Tracking

Auditory Perception
Figure-Ground
Memory (e.g., remembering a series of directions)
Discrimination

Tactile Perception
One-point Discrimination
Two-point Discrimination

The following perceptual-motor checklist can be used to screen participants suspected of having deficiencies and guide the instructor in determining which areas require more rigorous evaluation. For a more comprehensive listing of perceptual-motor test items, the reader is referred to excellent books by Lerch et al. (1974), Pyfer and Johnson (1983), Evans (1980), Williams (1983), and Sherrill (1986).

Perceptual-Motor Checklist

1. Does not demonstrate opposition of limbs during walking and/or running.

2. Fails to shift weight from one foot to the other when throwing.

3. Fails to imitate various body positions of evaluator or identify body parts on command.

4. Evidences flaccid muscle tone.

5. Is unable to use one body part without "overflow" into another.

6. Is unable to keep rhythm by clapping hands or tapping feet.

7. Cannot jump rope.

8. Is unable to coordinate the hands at the midline or cross the midline with one hand during activities.

9. Has difficulty identifying the right and left sides of the body.

10. Has difficulty distinguishing between vertical, horizontal, up, down, and other directions in space.

11. Cannot hop.

12. Has difficulty maintaining balance on one foot.

13. Has difficulty tying shoes, using scissors, manipulating small objects.

14. Has difficulty staying between lines.

15. Cannot discriminate tactually between different textures, shapes, and sizes.

16. Fails to maintain eye contact with moving objects.

17. Bumps into things; misjudges locations when moving to them. Is unable to move between or through objects.

18. Fails to match geometric shapes to one another (visually).

19. Cannot recognize letters and numbers.

20. Cannot distinguish between foreground and background in a picture.

21. Has difficulty catching balls.

22. Has difficulty walking on the balance beam.

Adapted from Sherrill, 1986

Perceptual-Motor Skill Progressions

Perceptual-motor skills generally refer to a person's ability to receive, interpret, and respond appropriately to a sensory stimuli. A comprehensive program to enhance perceptual-motor skills should provide activities involving the visual, auditory, tactile, and proprioceptive (vestibular and kinesthetic) senses.

A perceptual-motor program may be useful for remediating many neurologic dysfunctions: brain trauma, learning disabilities, mental retardation, aphasia, cerebral palsy, multiply sclerosis, and Parkinson's disease. The following lists of exercises have been employed with adults who evidence perceptual-motor deficiencies.

Balance Progressions

Balance is a skill underlying nearly every static and dynamic posture which requires the body to be stabilized against the pull of gravity. The physical management of the participant with impaired balance should be progressive in design. Developmentally, balance proceeds in a "cephalo-caudal" pattern. Stability is acquired in the neck region first and then proceeds downward (i.e., neck before shoulders; trunk before lower extremities). More specifically, balance activities should progress in the following sequence:

1. Rolling supine to prone and prone to supine.
2. Sitting with assistance.
3. Sitting without assistance.
4. Balancing with 4-point, 3-point, and 2-point stances.
5. Kneeling balance with a 2-point stance.
6. Standing balance with assistance (static).
7. Standing balance without assistance (static).
8. Standing balance with assistance (dynamic).
9. Standing balance without assistance (dynamic).
10. Ambulation training.
11. Training in ascending and descending stairs, ramps, and curbs.

Remember, when the participant is relearning a psycho-motor activity, break the skill down into small components, give clear instructions, provide proper demonstration, and provide corrective feedback. Watch for orthostatic hypotension when bringing an individual from a lying position to a seated one.

Activities for Developing
Static and Dynamic Balance

Supine to Prone Roll to Left Using Right Arm.

1. While supine, participant reaches across body with right arm and grasps side of mat and swings right leg if possible.
2. While supine, participant places right arm on mat at waist level, pushing and swing right leg to assist.

To Roll Right Using Right Arm

1. While supine, participant reaches for right edge of mat with right arm and grasps and pulls.
2. While supine, participant grasps upper portion of mat with right arm and pulls hard.

To Roll Left with Use of Right Leg

1. While supine, instruct participant to flex and adduct leg at knee joint and place foot on mat at midline of body and thrust vigorously while extending at both hip and knee.
2. While supine, flex and adduct at knee, swinging leg across body with enough momentum to rotate trunk.

Prone to Supine Using Right Arm to Turn Left

1. While prone, participant places right hand on mat with arm flexed/abducted and extends arm forcefully.
2. While prone, participant places right hand on mat with arm flexed/adducted and thrusts forcefully to a supine position.

Using Right Leg to Turn Left

While prone, raise the right leg backwards, swinging it in such a fashion to pull the person to his back.

Supine on Mat (or in bed)

1. Roll form back to front, and reverse in one smooth, continuous movement.
2. Roll from right side to left, hold for 2 seconds, and reverse with proper momentum so as not to land on back or front side.

Long-Sitting Position on Mat (Can be done in bed, chair, or on mat with support, as needed.)

1. Lean from side to side, using palms to retain balance.
2. Work up to leaning as far as possible with no arm support.
3. Resisted: Participant attempts to maintain upright position while assistant slowly applies pressure forward, backward, to right and left sides, and in rotation right and left. The assistant should hold each of these resistances for about 5 seconds each. Eventually, the assistant can give gentle pushes in the same directions while the participant attempts to maintain balance.
4. Participant attempts to bring right finger to nose. Repeat with left. Facing the assistant, the participant attempts to touch the right fingers to the assistant's right shoulder. Repeat with left.

Bridges

1. While in hook-lying position, participant elevates buttocks off the mat. Assistant may need to straddle the participant to keep the knees together and assist in elevating buttocks off mat.
2. If participant can perform this maneuver independently, assistant can provide resistance at the anterior superior iliac spines (ASIS), attempting to push buttocks back down to mat or side to side. Participant resists and attempts to maintain each position for about 5 seconds each.

4-Point Stance on Mat (on hands and knees)

Increase holding time in this position. Assistant may need to straddle participant and spot.

3-Point Stance on Mat

While on hands and knees, have participant raise and hold requested extremities (e.g., right arm, left arm).

2-Point Stance on Mat

While on hands and knees, have participant support body weight on two extremities while raising any combination of two (e.g., right arm with left leg).

Crawling Forward/Backward

Assistant kneels behind participant and assists participant with crawling by moving arms and legs as needed. Once the participant can maneuver forward and backward, teach participant to go right and left.

NOTE
This activity is precluded for those with joint trauma (i.e., knee and shoulder pain or inflammation).

Kneeling on Mat

Kneeling is more difficult because it raises the center of gravity and the base of support is smaller. The participant should be taught to rise to the kneeling position from the prone position. Eventually the participant is taught to rise from a kneeling position to a standing position.

The assistant generally spots from the front of the participant. As balance improves, the assistant can spot from behind. Once the participant can master a skill independently, a mirror should be placed in front of the participant. The participant should practice leaning right and left, forward and backward, successfully recovering balance each time.

Assisted Kneeling

The participant is assisted to a kneeling position. The participant then places the hands on the assistant's shoulders for support. The assistant may also need to stabilize at hips, trunk, or shoulders.

Resisted Kneeling

1. Participant should be able to balance on both knees, unassisted, for as long as possible.
2. Facing the participant, the assistant places his/her hands on the ASIS and attempts to push the participant backward. The participant should resist for approximately 5 seconds.
3. The assistant gently eases up on the pressure and slides the right hand around posteriorly. From this position, the assistant attempts to rotate the trunk to the participant's right. The participant should resist for 5 seconds and maintain the face forward position.
4. The assistant eases up on the pressure and slowly slides the left hand around posteriorly. From this position, the assistant attempts to pull the participant forward. The participant should resist for about 5 seconds, maintaining the upright posture.
5. The assistant eases up on the pressure and slowly slides the right hand anteriorly to the ASIS. From this position, the assistant attempts to rotate the trunk to the participant's left. The participant should resist for 5 seconds and maintain the face forward position.
6. Placing both hands on the ASIS, the assistant should attempt to push the participant to the side or at a diagonal. The participant should resist for 5 seconds, maintaining an upright posture.

Knee Walking

1. Walk forward, to each side, and backwards on knees with or without assistance.
2. Gradually increase distance.
3. Rock side-to-side in a rhythmic fashion.
4. Balance on one knee only.

Kneeling to Standing

1. Participant faces stall bars in supported kneeling position. Standing behind the participant, the assistant will place one hand on the shoulder and the other on the hip of participant. Ask the participant to position strong leg (flexed and slightly abducted) under body and extend with leg while pulling with strong arm.
2. Eventually the participant should be taught to come to standing position without use of stall bars.

Standing in Parallel Bars

1. Increase time for standing stationary (both supported and unsupported).
2. Add swaying by shifting weight from side to side, gradually widening the base of support.
3. Place one foot forward and one foot back to sway forward and back. Switch positions of the feet. If one foot is more affected, keep that one in front first.
4. All of the above can be performed with the eyes closed.
5. Resisted Balancing: See resisted balance activities under Resisted Kneeling. Perform same sequence in a standing position. Use both foot positions (i.e., side-by-side and forward-back).

Standing Static Balance in Parallel Bars

1. With arms abducted out to sides, participant attempts to balance on one leg. The other leg should be flexed at the knee and adducted at hip. This position is called a stork stand. As balance improves, hands can be moved to hips and then placed across the chest. The stork stand should be performed with the eyes closed as well.
2. Have participant perform these static positions on a balance beam.

Tilt Boards

1. Have participant begin with a wide base of support and progress to a narrow base.
2. Increase time on the tilt board.

Dynamic Balance

1. Have participant step over low objects placed on the floor. Use a mirror to allow participant to observe. Other variations include crossing leg over the midline while walking sideways.
2. Have participant walk a straight line marked on the floor with a spotter.
3. Have participant walk heel-to-toe on the balance beam. Practice forward, back, sideways. Always have a spotter present. Vary the width of the balance beam.
4. Have participant walk heel-to-toe on a circle marked on the floor with a spotter.

5. Have participant ascend and descend ramps and stairs. Step up stairs with the stronger leg first. Step down the stairs with the weaker leg first.
6. Have participant practice vertical jumps.
7. Have participant practice horizontal jumps (standing broad jump). Progress to taking successive jumps.
8. Have participant practice hopping on both right and left feet. Progress to hopping across room.

Activities for Developing Kinesthetic Awareness
(body awareness, laterality, bilateral coordination)

A prerequisite to the development of gross motor coordination is kinesthesis, or awareness of one's body in space. A simple test for up, down, right, left, forward, backward, and sideways may be given to determine the starting level for the individual. The following activities are designed to increase the individual's body awareness, laterality, and bilateral coordination.

Identification of Body Parts

1. Touch body parts one by one in response to one-word commands. For example: elbow, wrist, chin.
2. Upon command, touch two body parts simultaneously.
3. Touch five body parts in the same sequence as they are called by the assistant.
4. Repeat all of the above with eyes closed.

Right-Left Discrimination

1. Use the right hand to touch parts named on the right side.
2. Use the right hand to touch parts named on the left side. (This involves crossing the midline and should be more difficult than the previous task).
3. Use the left hand to touch parts named on the left side.
4. Use the left hand to touch parts named on the right side.
5. Given opportunities to touch body parts of a partner who is facing the participant:
   a. Use right hand to touch body parts on the right side of the partner.
   b. Use right hand to touch body parts on the left side of the partner.

Imitation of Postures/Movements

Have the participant imitate the arm and leg movements of the assistant in the sequence outlined on the next page:

Imitate Bilateral Movements

1. Move both arms apart and together while legs remain stationary.
2. Move both legs apart and together while arms remain stationary.
3. Move all four limbs apart and together simultaneously.
4. Move any three limbs apart and together while the fourth limb remains stationary.

Imitate Unilateral Movements

1. Move the right arm and right leg apart and together simultaneously while the left limbs remain stationary.
2. Move the left arm and leg apart and together simultaneously while the right limbs remain stationary.

Cross-lateral movements

1. Move the right arm and left leg apart and together simultaneously while the other limbs remain stationary.
2. Move the left arm and right leg apart and together simultaneously while the other limbs remain stationary.

Given opportunities to imitate arm movements of the assistant as described on the following page, have participant start and stop both arms simultaneously WITHOUT verbal instruction or mirroring.

Other Mat Exercises (Supine)

1. Lift right knee and intercept it with the right palm. Repeat to the left side.
2. Lift right knee and intercept it with the left palm. Repeat for the left knee and right palm.
3. With one leg raised, have the participant "write" numbers, letters, and names in the air with the foot.

4-Point Stance (On hands and knees)

1. Bring the right knee to touch right wrist. Repeat to the left side.
2. Bring the right knee to touch left wrist. Repeat with the left knee and right wrist.

Sitting (Work up to standing)

These activities are to be mirrored started with fingertips touching shoulders.
1. Extend arms overhead, then bring back to shoulders.
2. Reach both arms forward, then bring back to shoulders.
3. Stretch both arms out to side, then back to shoulders.
4. Repeat entire sequence 5-10 times, gradually increasing the speed. Eventually, have participant perform without mirroring the teacher.
5. Starting with arms down by the side, move the right hand to the right shoulder. Repeat to the left side.

Perceptual-Motor Games

Activity	Objective	Description
Move It	Directionality	Hop to right; skip to left, etc.
Bean Bag Toss & Catch	Laterality, Flexibility	Toss back up and catch over shoulder, under leg, etc.
Stone Walk	Motor Planning Laterality, Directionality, Balance	Place #'s on sheets of paper on ground. Give verbal or written directions of how to go through sequence.
Bean Bag Toss	Hand-Eye Coordination Laterality	Throw bags at target with assigned point value; stress proper throwing techniques.
Step and Walk	Visual-Motor Coordination, Dynamic Balance	Step over objects of various heights and widths.
Name Body Parts	Body Awareness	Touch specific body parts.
Crisscross Walk	Bilateral Coordination	Step across line with each leg.
Ball Bounce in Hoops	Eye-Hand Coordination	Bounce ball once in hoop #1. Bounce twice in hoop #2.
Jump and Turn	Directionality, Body Awareness, Dynamic balance	Jump and turn to specific angle or direction requested.
Walk and Dribble	Eye-Hand Coordination Spatial Awareness	Walk around course of cones while maintaining ball control.
Walk and Toss	Dynamic Balance Eye-Hand Coordination Tactile Awareness	While walking a straight line on balance beam, throw nerf ball at target.
Roll It	Laterality, Body Awareness	Roll ball up and down leg, around body, through legs. Emphasis on concepts of up and down, in, out.
Bounce It	Gross Motor	Bounce ball to assistant using one arm and two arms. Bounce ball to designated heights.
Throw It	Gross Motor	See above.
Cross It	Tactile Awareness Kinesthetic Awareness	Have various objects of different sizes, weights, and textures. Have participant find similar object from inside of surprise box.
Pick It	Fine Motor, Eye-Hand	Fill pan with small objects. Use a tweezer to pick objects up.
Listen & Do	Following Directions	Participant imitates the actions of assistant who puts hands on head, etc. Have participant follow spoken word while assistant touches unrelated body parts.
Cats in the Sand	Crossing Midline	Participant responds to directions for movements. Example: Move right arm and left leg while lying supine.

Fine Motor Tasks

Fine motor tasks usually refer to those involving use of the hands and fingers. Prehension and opposition are two commonly used terms when referring to tasks of this nature. Prehension refers to the ability to grasp an object with the fingers, while opposition refers to the ability to oppose any of the fingers with the thumb.

The following exercises emphasize fine motor coordination. Fine motor activities are generally harder to perform than gross motor.

1. Make a fist and then extend the fingers completely. Keep moving as fast as possible. Try to perform with one palm facing up and the other palm facing down. Reverse directions of palms for each hand. Try to perform with one fist open and one closed simultaneously.
2. With fingers extended, abduct and adduct together simultaneously. Try abducting and adducting fingers one at a time. Do one and then both hands at the same time.
3. Make a circle with each individual finger.
4. With the dominant hand, touch the thumb to each finger of that hand individually. Proceed from the index finger to the little finger, and reverse the direction back up to the index finger again. Work up to using both hands at the same time. Eventually, increase the speed and perform with the eyes closed.
5. With arm stretched out in front, touch the index finger to nose, and to a real (dot on board) or imaginary point straight ahead. Repeat as fast and accurately as possible within 30 seconds. Later, try the same with the eyes closed. Use the dominant arm before the non-dominant arm.
6. Try to touch the right index finger to the nose while extending the left arm out to the side. Alternate by touching the nose with the left index finger while simultaneously extending the right arm out to the side.

Study Questions / Learning Activities

1. Diagram and label the perceptual-motor process.

2. Using a partner, perform the entire progression of static and dynamic balance exercises described in this chapter.

3. Devise a critierion-referenced test for static balance (10 items or less) and administer the test first to a partner, then an adult with balance deficits. Design an exercise program for static balance, based on the assessment.

4. Devise a perceptual-motor game and explain its purpose.

References

Cratty, B. J. (1986). *Perceptual and motor development in infants and children.* Englewood Cliffs, NJ: Prentice-Hall.

Evans, J. R. (1980). *They have to be carefully taught.* American Alliance for Health, Physical Education, Recreation and Dance, Stock Number 245-26904.

Lerch, H. A., Becker, J. E., Ward, B. M., & Nelson, J. A. (1974). *Perceptual-motor learning - theory and practice.* Palo Alto, CA: Peek Publications.

Pyfer, J., & Johnson, R. (1984). *Adapted physical education. Evaluation and pro-gramming for students with handicapping conditions.* Topeka: Kansas State Department of Eduation.

Sherrill, C. (1986, 3rd ed.). *Adapted physical education and recreation.* Dubuque: Wm. C. Brown.

Werner, P., & Rini, L. (1976). *Perceptual-motor development equipment.* New York: John Wiley & Sons.

Williams, H. (1983). *Perceptual and motor development.* Englewood Cliffs, NJ: Prentice-Hall.

CHAPTER 11

Assessment and Programming for Posture

Assessment of Posture

Before assessing postural deviations, it is necessary to have an understanding of possible underlying causes of deviations. This knowledge will assist in determining whether medical referral or exercise prescription is the more appropriate intervention. A thorough discussion of each deviation may be found in Sherrill (1986).

To conduct a posture evaluation, the adapted physical educator utilizes a posture screen or plumb line in conjunction with observations. A plumb line is a thick piece of rope suspended from the ceiling with a weighted end (weight should not touch the floor). A schematic of a posture screen may be found in Appendix C of this manual. If pictures are used, the participant should be photographed in anterior, posterior, and lateral views. The participant should be barefoot, wearing a swimsuit, and have the hair pulled back behind the ears. If a large group has to be screened at the same time, stations should be set up with individuals rotating to each station.

Description of the Posture Evaluation

Strength

Abdominals

Weak abdominal musculature has been implicated in the occurrence of low back pain. No norm-referenced test exists which purely measures abdominal strength - current tests also activate the hip flexors. A modified sit-up test with norms for those between the ages of 5 to 17 years can be found in the AAHPERD Health Related Physical Fitness Test Manual (see reference at end of this chapter). This exercise partially eliminates the action of the hip flexors during movement. The score is recorded as the number of sit-ups performed in one minute. Other abdominal exercises can be found in Chapter 6.

Flexibility

Chest and Shoulders

Participant assumes a hook-lying position. Keeping the low back pressed to the floor (assistant should check by placing a hand between the lumbar region and floor), the participant extends the arms overhead and presses the back of the arms and hands to the floor. Elbows must remain locked at all times.

Scoring: Within Normal Limits (WNL) — contact of dorsum of hands with the floor. Limitation of Motion (LOM) — contact of fingers only or cannot make contact with floor without arching the low back.

Spine and Hip Extensors

See Sit and Reach test in Chapter 7 on page 95.

Scoring: Record the number of inches or centimeters reached by the fingertips.

Hip Flexors

See Thomas test in Chapter 7 on page 96.

Scoring: WNL — if thigh remains flat on the table.
LOM — if thigh lifts upward. Estimate angle between leg and table. *Note: If thigh rotates outward or inward, rotators are tight. Indicate on evaluation form.*

Orthopedic Evaluation

Foot Examination

Note pes planus, pes cavus, Achilles flare, hallux valgus, overlapping toes, hammer toes, corns, and calluses.

Flexible Pes Planus

Involves measurement of the navicular. The instructor first marks the farthest medial projection of the navicular with a dot or short line parallel to the floor. The participant is then asked to place the foot on a flat surface without bearing weight on it, and the instructor measures the distance from the supporting surface to the mark on the navicular bone. The participant then stands on the foot and the height of the mark is again measured.

Scoring: Record the degree of fluctuation of the navicular between weight-bearing and non-weight bearing. If greater than 1/4 inch, pes planus is indicated.

Scoliosis Check

See "Procedures for Spinal Screening" in this chapter. Scoliosis screening is usually performed on children in elementary and secondary grades since treatment is very difficult after bone growth is complete. However, older participants experiencing low back pain may benefit from this type of screening to determine the nature of their pain.

Anterior View

Draw a plumb line from a point equidistant between the medial malleoli and extending perpendicular to the floor, bisecting the body (see following illustration).
Note any of the following:

1. **Head Twist** (torticollis) or Head Tilt - Check the evenness of the earlobes and indicate left or right drop.
2. **Shoulder Level** - Note evenness of acromion processes and indicate left or right drop.
3. **Linea Alba** - Indicate a left or right shift.
4. **Anterior Superior Iliac Spines** (hip) — Note evenness and indicate left or right drop.
5. **Leg Alignment** - Beginning at the center of the knee, draw a line perpendicular to the floor.
   a) Internal or external rotation at the hip. The knee and foot both point outward or inward.
   b) Internal tibial torsion. The patella faces inward when the feet are together, pointing forward.
   c) Genu valgum (knock knees). Note the space between the medial malleoli when knees are touching.
   d) Genu varum (bow legs). Note the space between the femoral condyles when the feet are together.
   e) Pronation. The big toe (first metatarsal) falls lateral to the plumb line drawn from the center of the knee.

Plumb Lines and Anatomical References for Anterior View

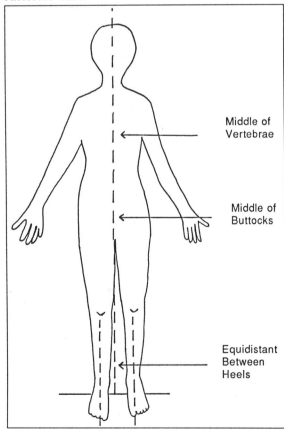

Middle of Vertebrae

Middle of Buttocks

Equidistant Between Heels

Lateral View

Draw a plumb line beginning with a point one and 1/2 inches anterior to center of the lateral malleolus and proceed upward, perpendicular to the floor. In ideal posture, the plumb line should pass through the following fixed check points: center of the knee (behind the patella), center of the hip (greater trochanter), center of the shoulder (acromion process), and through the earlobe (tragus). Postural abnormalities are based on the deviation (forward or backward) from this line (see following illustration).

Plumb Line and Anatomical References for Lateral View

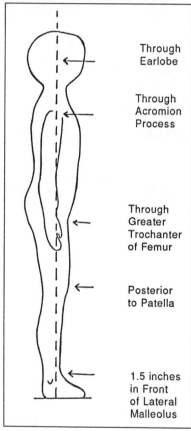

Through Earlobe

Through Acromion Process

Through Greater Trochanter of Femur

Posterior to Patella

1.5 inches in Front of Lateral Malleolus

Note any of the following:

1. **Body Lean** — Indicate whether forward or backward.
2. **Head** — Considered forward if the earlobe is in front of the acromion process.
3. **Shoulders** — Considered forward if acromion process is in front of plumb line.
4. **Kyphosis** — Excessive flexion in the thoracic spine. Check for structural kyphosis in Adam's position.
5. **Lordosis** — Excessive hyperextension in lumbar spine
6. **Ptosis** — Abdominal protrusion. Abdominals should not extend beyond a line drawn down from the sternum.
7. **Genu Recurvatum** (hyperextended knees) — Patella falls behind plumb line.

Posterior View

Winged Scapula (protrusion of the inferior border — Indicate whether right or left.

Procedures for Spinal Screening

(adapted from Children's Hospital, San Diego, California)

First

Ask if there is a history of scoliosis in the family.

Second

Look at participant's back while he/she is standing. Ask yourself:

1. Are earlobes level?
2. Are shoulders (acromion processes) the same level?
3. Are inferior borders of the scapulae the same level?
4. Are arms the same distance from the body?
5. Are trunk contours the same on both sides of body?
6. Are hips level?
7. Are poplitial creases level?

The above are pieces of a puzzle. A positive finding in any of the above may be a normal variant or may indicate scoliosis. The next check is perhaps the most important.

Third

The participant bends forward about 90 degrees with hands together, feet together, and head down as if diving into a pool (Adam's position). View the participant from the back. Ask yourself:
Is one side of the thoracic or lumbar spine higher than the other?

Fourth

The participant bends forward as above, but view the participant from the front. Ask yourself: Is one side of the thoracic or lumbar spine higher than the other?

Fifth

Take a quick look at the side view of the participant as a check for kyphosis. Ask yourself: Is the curve even or does it peak?

With children and teenagers, a medical referral is warranted if an asymmetry is noted in Adam's position, indicating possible structural scoliosis. Adults are generally not referred because bone growth is complete. Exercises can be prescribed to combat pain and loss of flexibility.

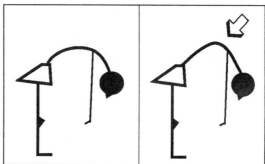

Posture Exercises

Forward Head

Starting Position	Movement	Purpose
Neck Flattener	1. Press back of neck firmly to floor (feel contraction in both neck extensors and flexors.) 2. Hold 5 seconds. 3. REPS:____ SETS:____	1. To strengthen neck flexors and extensors.
Revolving Neck Flattener	1. Press back of neck firmly to floor. 2. Slowly turn the head from side to side. 3. REPS:____ SETS:____	1. To strengthen neck flexors, extensors, and rotators.
Side Head Lift	1. Turn head to right side, right ear to floor. 2. Keeping head in this position, lift toward ceiling. 3. Hold 5 seconds. 4. REPS:____ SETS:____	1. To strengthen neck rotators.
Military Tuck	1. Pull chin and head backward as far as possible (keep eye on a horizontal plane). Do not tilt head. 2. Hold 5 seconds. 3. REPS:____ SETS:____	1. To strengthen neck flexors and extensors.

Forward Shoulders/Kyphosis

Butterfly	1. Clasp Hands over low back. 2. Attempt to draw elbows together. 3. Hold 10 seconds. 4. REPS:____ SETS:____	1. To strengthen muscles which retract the shoulders and adduct the scapula. (rhomboids, trapezius)
Prone Lift Arms Overhead	1. Lift arms only from floor (elbows extended). 2. When capable, lift arms and head only. 3. When capable, lift arms, head, and shoulders only (do not arch low back). May be performed with upper back over table. 4. Hold 5 seconds. 5. REPS:____ SETS:____	1. To strengthen muscles which retract the shoulders and adduct the scapula. 2. To strengthen upper bac extensors.

Starting Position	Movement	Purpose
Wall Lean	1. Face corner of room, one hand on either wall at shoulder height. 2. Incline body toward the corner, bending elbows (heels on floor). 3. Hold 10 seconds. 4. REPS:____ SETS:____	1. To stretch anterior chest muscles (pectorals).
Prone Lift Arms Extended Sideward	1. Pinch shoulder blades together. 2. Raise arms slightly from mat. 3. Raise head from mat (chin in). 4. Hold for 5 seconds. 5. REPS:____ SETS:____	1. To strengthen muscles which retract the shoulders and adduct the scapula. 2. To improve alignment of upper back and head.
Sitting Hand Slide	1. Hands placed on low back. 2. Slowly slide hands up back attempting to bring elbows together. 3. REPS:____ SETS:____	1. To stretch anterior chest muscles. 2. To strengthen muscles which retract the shoulders and adduct the scapula
Towel Stretch	1. Raise towel overhead. Hold for 10 seconds. 2. Lower towel obliquely across back. Hold for 10 seconds. 3. Reverse position. 4. REPS:____ SETS:____	1. To strengthen muscles which retract the shoulders and adduct the scapula. 2. To strengthen external rotators of shoulders. 3. To stretch anterior chest muscles.
Shoulder Stretch	1. Allow gravity to hyperflex the shoulder joint. 2. It may be necessary to flex the knees slightly if the hamstrings are tight. 3. Hold 10 to 30 seconds. 4. REPS:____	1. To stretch the anterior chest muscles and internal rotators of shoulders.
Bent Arm Press Supine	1. Elbows flexed, arms in external rotation. 2. Press back with the back of the hand against a hard surface, keeping low back on floor. 3. Hold for 10 seconds. 4. REPS:____ SETS:____	1. To strengthen external rotators of the shoulders.

Starting Position	Movement	Purpose
Push Up	1. Tighten abdominal and gluteal muscles. 2. Bend elbows, lowering body to floor. 3. Raise the body. Do not bend at the waist. 4. REPS:____ SETS:____	1. To strengthen the shoulder girdle muscles, especially the serratus anterior. 2. To assist in correcting winged scapula. 3. Activate the abdominals and gluteals.
Prone Flies	1. Slowly raise dumbbells out to side and above level of body. 2. Arms may be slightly bent. 3. Repeat 10 times. 4. REPS:____ SETS:____	1. To strengthen the muscles which retract shoulders and adduct the scapula.
Shoulder Flexion with Pulleys	1. Keeping arms straight, slowly lift pulleys overhead. 2. Do not arch lower back. 3. Repeat 10 times. 4. REPS:____ SETS:____	1. To strengthen upper back extensors (trapezius).
Backward Shoulder Rolls	1. Rotate both shoulders **slowly** in circles up (to ears) and backward. 2. REPS:____ SETS:____	1. Strengthen muscles which retract the shoulders and adduct the scapula.
Horizontal Ladder	1. Travel along one side of ladder. 2. Travel with one hand on each side of ladder. 3. Travel across ladder, one rung at a time. 4. Travel across ladder, skipping one rung each time. 5. REPS:____ SETS:____	1. To stretch the muscles of the shoulder and spine.

Lower Extremities

Heel Cord Stretch Standing at arms length from wall, body inclined slightly forward, back flat feet in-toed slightly.	1. Hands on wall shoulder high and shoulder width apart, elbows slightly bent. Bend arms until chest nearly touches the wall. Keep body in straight line, keep heels on the floor. 2. Progression: From starting position, move backward about an inch at a time keeping heels on the floor. 3. Heel cord stretch board with back flattened against the wall may be used as an advanced exercise. 4. Hold for 30 seconds. 5. REPS:____	1. To stretch heel cord and back of leg. Beneficial in pes planus, pronation.

Starting Position	Movement	Purpose
Ankle Stretch Standing on lower rung of stall bar, feet slightly in-toed and weight on balls of feet. Grasp an upper rung for support to aid in balancing.	1. Raise on toes as high as possible. 2. Lower body to stretch heel cord as heels are slowly below the level of the support. Be sure weight is on the outer margin of feet at all times and stand tall throughout the exercise. 3. Hold stretch for 30 seconds. 4. REPS:____	1. To stretch anterior tibial and calf muscles. 2. Beneficial in pes planus and pronation, fractures of the ankles, post-operative repair, and following the use of a cast on the limb.
Foot Supinator Sitting Tall	1. Cross leg so the ankle of right foot rests across left knee, keeping the foot at right angles to the right leg and turning the sole of the foot upward. 2. Place left palm on medial border of right foot. Attempt to push the right foot downward (pronation). Resist and hold the right foot insupination. 3. Hold for 10 seconds. 4. REPS:____ SETS:____	1. Strengthens invertors, supinators of foot. 2. Beneficial in pes planus and pronation.
Frog Kick Sitting on floor with legs extended. Place hands on mat behind buttocks with fingers pointed forward.	1. Fully flex the knees and place the soles of the feet together. 2. Then with the heels on the floor and the feet perpendicular (toes pointing upward) to the floor, extend the legs keeping the soles of the feet together. 3. Hold and stretch for 10 seconds. 4. Return slowly. 5. REPS:____ SETS:____	1. Strengthens invertors of the foot. 2. Beneficial in pes planus, pronation, and tibial torsion.
Knee Flexion **(with boot)** Lying face down with a bootstrapped on the foot, leg and ankle extended.	1. Raise lower leg to vertical position, hold, slowly return. 2. Do not bend knee more than 90 degrees.	1. Strengthens hamstrings (knee flexors). 2. Beneficial in genu recurvatum.

Study Questions / Learning Activities

1. Assess your posture (anterior, posterior, and lateral views) with a partner or use a mirror.

2. Develop an exercise program to correct any deviations you might have.

3. Note and record the characteristic postures of different age groups. For example, compare toddlers to teenagers and young adults to seniors. What differences do you see in posture of the head, trunk, stomach, and legs of these groups?

References

AAHPERD Health Related Fitness Test. American Alliance for Health, Physical Education, Recreation and Dance.

Auxter, D., & Pyfer, J. (1985). *Principles and methods of adapted physical education and recreation.* St. Louis: Times Mirror/Mosby College.

Kendall, H. O., & Kendall, F. P. (1968). Developing and maintaining good posture. *Journal of Physical Therapy, 48*(4).

Lowman, C. L., & Young, C. H. (1960). *Postural fitness.* Philadelphia: Lea & Febiger.

Sherrill, C. (1986, 3rd ed.). *Adapted physical education and recreation.* Dubuque: Wm. C. Brown.

CHAPTER 12

Assessment and Programming for Adapted Aquatics

Adapted Aquatics — Hydrogymnastics

Hydrogymnastics is an individualized exercise program performed in the water. The purpose of Hydrogymnastics is to utilize the water as a therapeutic modality to habilitate individuals with disabilities.

The adapted aquatic setting provides the participant with the opportunity to do activities that may not be possible on land. Hydrogymnastics can be enjoyed by persons with most disabilities, but it is especially well-suited to people with orthopedic/joint limitations, obesity, ambulation difficulties, and low-back syndrome. There are a few conditions, however, where an adapted aquatics program would be contraindicated, such as severe hypertension or hypotension, cardiac conditions, infective skin disorders, and incontinence.

During an adapted aquatic session, the participant can experience both success and mobility due in part to the buoyancy of the water. Buoyancy neutralizes the effects of gravity. Water supports the individual and he/she will notice a sensation of weightlessness. This feature allows the participant to move more freely and with less energy expenditure than when on land.

One advantage of performing exercises in the pool is the ability to modify resistance easily. As the participant's strength increases, simple changes in the speed of movement or in the placement of the extremities against the line of movement will increase the resistance. If further resistance is desired, the incorporation of hand paddles, kickboards, or swim fins while performing the exercises will generate significant resistance.

Many people prefer Hydrogymnastics because it occurs in a warm pool (92-93 degrees F). It is believed that warm water decreases pain and induces relaxation. With this decreased pain, many participants can see noticeable improvements in their range of motion. It is a well established fact that warm water is a vasodilator which increases peripheral blood flow. An important physiological point to remember is that as one enters the water, cutaneous vessels constrict momentarily causing a rise in blood pressure. However, during immersion, the arterioles will dilate, possibly causing the participant to feel light-headed.

The benefits of Hydrogymnastics are many and can be categorized into three areas: physiological, social, and psychological. The following listings were adapted from the American Red Cross Instructor's Manual.

Physiological Benefits

1. Increases muscular strength and endurance.
2. Facilitates improvement in flexibility.
3. Enhances peripheral circulation and provides opportunities to address cardiovascular endurance.
4. Provides an exercise setting where respiration and metabolic rates are elevated.
5. Allows the participant an opportunity to develop gross motor coordination skills.
6. Will induce relaxation in a warm water environment.

Psychological Benefits

A participant's self-image and confidence may be boosted. Within the water, the disability is less noticeable. The participant is less handicapped in the water. Therefore, the water environment provides an opportunity where the participant with physical limitations is more like his/her able-bodied peers.

Social Benefits

1. Provides an enjoyable activity. The time spent in the pool may be the only time when joints and muscles don't hurt.
2. Offers an opportunity to socialize. The pool is a place where persons, both able-bodied and disabled, can share and compete equally.
3. Provides a recreational opportunity. Within an aquatic session, the participant with a disability can participate in vigorous physical activities not possible on land.
4. Sets up healthy recreational opportunities. From learning to swim, the student can branch out to other water activities, such as sailing, water skiing, or snorkling.

In order to have your participant derive the aforementioned benefits, your comprehensive adapted aquatics program should include:

1. Therapeutic exercises to develop muscular strength and endurance, flexibility, and cardiovascular fitness.
2. Water safety skills.
3. Instruction of swimming skills, modified to the capabilities of the participant.
4. Gait training, employing the use of weighted canes, walkers, etc. Participants with paralysis of the lower extremities should wear socks to prevent scrapes.
5. Lap swimming to provide opportunity for cardiovascular training.
6. Instruction in games and sports to enhance psycho-motor skills, as well as fostering greater interaction and sportsmanship.

Entrance and exit into the pool can present a potentially difficult situation for participants with severe impairments. It is essential that assistants be present both on the deck and in the pool as lifeguards, assistants, and spotters.

For participant s who will be entering and exiting the pool with the use of the ladder, it is important to teach them to always face the ladder. This method allows for greater control and safety.

If your program includes participants who have incurred a cerebrovascular accident, it is recommended that you pad the rungs of the ladder to prevent bruising of the shins. Participants with hemiparesis should lead with the weak leg going down the ladder as they enter the pool. When exiting from the pool, the participant should lead with the strong leg up the ladder (remember the adage: up with the good; down with the bad).

If the participant is unable to maneuver down the ladder, the decision of using a Hoyer lift or a two-man transfer must be made. it is important to ask the participant which method is preferred, because many persons with disabilities do not like the Hoyer lift. This method tends to attract attention to the participant, and it is uncomfortable to sit in a wet, cold lift while waiting to be placed in the water. Before deciding which method will be used, it is essential to take into consideration the weight of the participant and the strength of the assistants.

Generally, the two-man transfers are easily and safely accomplished when the assistants work as a team. Each assistant takes a position on either side of the participant. The assistants should employ the same techniques used in a typical two-man transfer (see Chapter 4 on page 48). Once the participant is on the deck, one assistant will stand behind the participant and grasp the forearms from under the axillas. The second assistant should be in the water guiding the participant into the pool. The second assistant should position his/her hands around the participant's waist.

When assisting the participant out of the pool with the two-man lift, utilize the buoyancy of the water by bouncing the participant several times before lifting. Extreme care should be taken so that the participant will not hit his/her tailbone on the deck after being pulled out of the water.

In addition, flotation devices should be placed in position prior to entering the water. In exiting the pool, this procedure should be reversed.

Teaching Suggestions

The following techniques have proven useful when working with participants in a hydrogymnastic setting. These tips are categorized into two groups: (1) tips related to swim instruction; and (2) tips related to ambulation training and therapeutic exercise.

Swim Instruction Tips

1. Set up the situation so that the participant will succeed.
2. Teach the appropriate sequence of skills, dependent upon disability, motivational level, and interests.
3. For participants with hemiparesis, teach symmetric, bilateral, underwater recovery strokes first (e.g., elementary backstroke, breast-stroke).
4. Use flotation and swim aids as necessary. Try not to develop over-dependency on such equipment.

Hydrotherapy Tips

1. When teaching ambulation skills, make sure that the participant is sufficiently buoyant.
2. During gait training, do not allow participant to drag the feet on the bottom of the pool. Have participant wear socks or shoes to prevent scrapes.
3. It is recommended when teaching ambulation skills to have the assistant wear a face mask in order to observe leg movements.
4. "Draft" the weaker participants when practicing walking. This maneuver is accomplished when the assistant walks backwards to decrease the resistance of the water. Later, if additional resistance is desired, have the participant push a kickboard while walking.
5. The water is an excellent medium to teach the participant the techniques of self-range of motion.

Therapeutic Aquatic Exercises

Exercises for the Lower Extremities

Position: Standing with back or side to pool wall. Participant holds on to pool gutter.

1. Raise heels off the ground. Lower. Repeat 15 times.
2. With arms at side, stretch by slowly bending to the left. Repeat to the other side. Repeat 10 times each side.
3. Raise left knee to chest. Extend left leg straight out. Drop leg to starting position. Repeat with the left leg. Repeat 10 times each leg.
4. Raise left foot as high as possible with leg straight. Swing foot and leg to left side. Recover to starting position by pulling left leg vigorously to right. Reverse to right leg. Repeat 10 times.

5. Raise left leg and clasp calf with both arms pulling to chest. Return to starting position. Repeat exercise with the right leg. Repeat 10 times.
6. With pool edge on right, stretch left arm out in front at shoulder height. Standing on tiptoes, swing left leg forwards and then backward.s Repeat for right leg. Repeat 10 times.
7. With pool edge on right, stretch left arm out to side. Circle the left leg. Repeat for right leg. Repeat 10 times.
8. With back to edge, bend left knee. Extend foot, then return to bent-knee position. Repeat for the right leg. Repeat 10 times.

Position: Holding on to gutter with back towards edge. Feet not touching the bottom of pool.

1. Bring knees to chest. Extend legs without the feet touching the bottom. Return to the starting position. Repeat 10 times.
2. With the legs extended, swing legs far apart. Bring legs together crossing left leg over right. Swing legs far apart. Bring legs together crossing right over left. Repeat 10 times.

Exercises for the Upper Extremities

Position: Standing facing the pool edge.

1. Standing approximately 12 inches from the wall with the shoulders under water, twist left and try to touch wall with both hands. Twist right and try to touch wall with both hands. Repeat 10 times.
2. With shoulders under water, stretch arms out in front at shoulder height. Swing them down together past the sides of the body and out behind. Swing back again the same way to starting positions. Repeat 15 times.
3. With shoulders under water, raise arms to shoulder height and flex elbows so hands touch each other, palms down in front of chest. Flap elbows up and down quickly. Repeat 20 times.
4. Stretch arms out in front and swing them around and as far behind as possible, keeping them at shoulder height. Return to the starting position. Repeat 20 times.
5. With shoulders under water, circle arms. Make small and large circles. Repeat 20 times.
6. With shoulders under water, bring arms towards ears in lateral direction, palms facing up. In returning, turn palms down. Repeat 20 times.
7. With shoulders under water, circle wrists in one direction, then switch to the other direction.
8. Make a fist, then extend fingers.

Assessment of Aquatic Skills

The following forms can be used to evaluate pre-, beginning, and advanced swim skills. The participant should be pretested and post-tested to determine improvements derived from the training program.

ADAPTED AQUATICS EVALUATION SHEET
TEST A: PRE-SWIMMING SKILLS

STUDENT'S NAME:_____

ADMISSION DATE:_____

Evaluator:_____Date:_____
Evaluator:_____Date:_____
Evaluator:_____Date:_____

                                                            Date Achieved

1. Enters water: with assistance   _____
                                    without assistance _____

2. Stands in waist/chest deep water: supported   _____
                                          unsupported _____

3. Walks forward in waist/chest deep water: supported   _____
                                              unsupported _____

4. Walks side-stepping in waist/chest   supported   _____
   deep water: unsupported _____

5. Walks backward in waist/chest   supported   _____
   deep water.   unsupported _____

6. Holds onto wall: with assistance   _____
                                    without assistance _____

7. Holds onto wall and traverses perimeter of pool   _____

8. Jumps up and down in chest   with assistance   _____
   deep water: without assistance _____

Comments:_____
_____
_____
_____

ADAPTED AQUATICS EVALUATION SHEET
TEST B: BEGINNER SWIM SKILLS

STUDENT'S NAME: _____

ADMISSION DATE: _____

Evaluator:_____   Date: _____
Evaluator:_____   Date: _____
Evaluator:_____   Date: _____

Date Achieved

1.	Puts face in water:	with assistance _____
		without assistance _____
2.	Blows bubbles:	with assistance _____
		without assistance _____
3.	Supine float:	with assistance _____
		without assistance _____
4.	Prone float:	with assistance _____
		without assistance _____
5.	Flutter kick-board or assist:	with assistance _____
		without assistance _____
6.	Supine float & recovery:	with assistance _____
		without assistance _____
7.	Prone float & recovery:	with assistance _____
		without assistance _____
8.	Glide-prone & supine:	with assistance _____
		without assistance _____
9.	Prone glide with kick:	with assistance _____
		without assistance _____
10.	Basic crawl stroke & breathing:	with assistance _____
		without assistance _____

ADAPTED AQUATICS EVALUATION SHEET
TEST B: BEGINNER SWIM SKILLS

continued

Date Achieved

11. Sculling-hands figure 8's: with assistance _____
                                             without assistance _____

12. Change position-prone to   with assistance _____
    supine: without assistance _____

13. Change position-supine to   with assistance _____
    prone: without assistance _____

14. Underwater swim: with assistance _____
                                           without assistance _____

15. Can perform symmetrial strokes:
    A)   sculling   yes___   no___
    B)   finning   yes___   no___
    C)   elementary backstroke
          arms only___   legs only___   combined arms and legs___
    D)   breast stroke
          arms only___   legs only___   combined arms and legs___

16. Can perform asymmetrial strokes:
    A)   crawl/free style
          arms only___   legs only___   combined arms and legs___

    B)   backstroke
          arms only___   legs only___   combined arms and legs___

17. Can breath when doing crawl stroke:
                                     with assistance _____
                                     without assistance _____

18. Retrieves object from bottom:
                              with assistance (2' depth) _____
                              without assistance (2' depth) _____
                              with assistance (3' depth) _____
                              without assistance (3' depth) _____

ADAPTED AQUATICS EVALUATION SHEET
TEST B: BEGINNER SWIM SKILLS

continued

___

Date Achieved

19.   Surface dives to bottom: assisted (5' depth)   _____
                                   unassisted (5' depth)   _____

20.   Jumps into deep water: assisted and is caught   _____
                                 unassisted and is caught   _____

21.   Jumps into deep water: assisted and swims to side   _____
                                 unassisted and swims to side   _____

22.   Changes direction: to left   _____
                                              to right   _____

23.   Changes position: horizontal plane, front to back   _____
                                            back to front   _____
                              vertical plane, front to back   _____
                                            back to front   _____

24.   Uses kickboard: with assistance   _____
                                 without assistance   _____

Comments: _____

_____

_____

_____

_____

_____

_____

_____

_____

_____

ADAPTED AQUATICS EVALUATION SHEET
TEST C: ADVANCED SWIM SKILLS

STUDENT'S NAME:_____

ADMISSION DATE:_____

Evaluator:_____Date:_____

Evaluator:_____Date:_____

Evaluator:_____Date:_____

TEST A Skills passed on (date):_____

TEST B Skills passed on (date):_____

Date Achieved

1. Bobs without pushing off bottom (6' depth)   _____

2. Crawl (C) stroke with out of water arm recovery:

    20'   _____

    40'   _____

3. Crawl stroke with breathing to the side:

    20'   _____

    40'   _____

4. Basic Backstroke (40')   _____

5. Racing Backstroke (RBS):   20'   _____

    40'   _____

6. Breast-stroke (BS):   20'   _____

    40'   _____

7. Side-stroke (SS):   20'   _____

    40'   _____

8. Head first dive: with assistance   _____

    without assistance   _____

9. Surface dive: 7' depth   _____

    9' depth   _____

10. Distance swim (30 minutes) with any stroke   _____

Comments:_____

_____

_____

_____

HYDROGYMNASTICS ASSESSMENT TOOL

STUDENT'S NAME:_____

PRE-TEST DATE:_____ POST-TEST DATE:_____

ABILITY TO SWIM ACROSS POOL?   Yes _____ No _____

Stroke Used_____

Crawl Stroke	+	o	-
Elementary Back	+	o	-
Side Stroke, lt.	+	o	-
Side Stroke, rt.	+	o	-
Breast Stroke	+	o	-
Butterfly	+	o	-
_____	+	o	-
_____	+	o	-

FLEXIBILITY:

Apley Scratch Test	rt.	up	yes	close	no
	lt.	up	yes	close	no
Straight Leg Raises	rt.	up	yes	close	no
	lt.	up	yes	close	no

MUSCULAR ENDURANCE:

Kickboard push #30   _____

Arm Circle #30   _____

Leg Flutters #30   _____

Knees to chest #30   _____

Jog across pool rate   _____ # of sec. & heart

Body composition   _____% _____%

ALTERNATES

_____   _____

_____   _____

Evaluator's Name_____ Date_____

Name_____ Date_____

Subjective, did the student show improvement:?_____

_____

_____

_____

Definition of Test Items on Hydrogymnastic Assessment Tool

Apley Scratch Test   See Apley Scratch Test under Active Range of Motion Tests in Chapter 7 on page 93.

Straight Leg Raises   Stand in the pool with the back to the wall. Raise the leg up as close to the surface of the water as possible.

Kickboard Push #30   Stand in the water with the kickboard held lengthwise. Push and pull kickboard as fast as possible for 30 seconds.

Arm Circle #30   Stand in the water with the arms abducted. Make large circles backwards for 30 seconds.

Leg Flutters #30   Holding onto the wall in a prone position, kick as fast as possible for 30 seconds.

Knees to Chest #30   Holding the edge of the pool with the back against the wall, bring the knees to the chest repeatedly for 30 seconds.

Jog Across Pool   In chest deep water, jog across pool as fast as possible. Measure the time it takes to cross the pool and note the heart rate.

Study Questions / Learning Activities

1. Which types of disabilities benefit most from the gentle water environment found in an adapted aquatics program?

2. List the physiological, psychological, and social benefits of an adapted aquatics program.

3. Visit an aquatics program for adults with disabilities such as the Arthoswim program. Note the types of disabilities, ages of participants, equipment, music (if any), teaching style and methods, and exercises performed. What conclusions can you draw about this type of program?

Reference

Knopf, K. G., Fleck, L., & Martin, M. (1992). *Water workout.* Winston Salem, NC: Hunter Textbooks.

13

Specific Disabilities

Acquired Brain Injury

One of the more challenging aspects of post-secondary adapted physical education is that of assessing and programming for persons with acquired brain injury (ABI). Few disabilities present such an impairment of cognitive, physical, psychosocial, and emotional functioning. While the deficits may loom large and often discourage adapted physical educators, a truly rewarding experience can be had as many of these individuals possess great potential for improvement.

Brain damage can be primary (impact) or secondary. Primary damage includes skull fractures, contusions of the gray matter, and diffuse white-matter lesions (Umphred, 1985). Secondary damage occurs after trauma has been introduced (as early as one hour after) and may involve brain swelling, intracranial hematoma, cerebral hypoxia, and ischemia. The resulting impairment does not depend on the cause of the lesion, but rather the location affected within the brain. Examples of traumatic and disease entities that clinically fall into the category of acquired brain injury and approximate the same symptoms include:

1. Traumatic Head Injury
   a. Closed head trauma
   b. Penetrating tissue wound
   c. Skull fractures
2. Cerebrovascular accident (stroke)
3. Ingestion of neurotoxic substances or drug overdoses
4. Brain tumors
5. Hypoxia (e.g., near-drowning
6. Infections of the brain

Sequelae and Complications	
Cognitive	Impairment of memory, attention span, reasoning, organizational thinking skills, spatial orientation, and information processing. Presence of perseveration.
Psycho-Motor	Involvement of neuromotor system. Impairment of balance, gross and fine motor coordination, and strength. Presence of primitive reflexes and abnormal muscle tone.
Linguistic	Impairment of expressive and receptive language, and related communication skills (aphasia and dysarthria).
Psycho-Social	Impulsivity, disinhibition, denial, poor social judgment, aggressiveness, emotional lability, untoward social behavior, irritability.
Sensory-Perceptual	Primary perceptual deficits, visual, auditory, tactile modalities.

In order to understand the sequelae of an individual with ABI, it is necessary to learn the basic functional components of the brain. The brain is the control center for all of the body's functions, including thinking, moving and breathing. It receives messages, interprets them, and then responds to them by enabling the person to speak, move, or show emotion. The brain is protected by the thick layer of skull and surrounded by cerebrospinal fluid which allows the brain to "float" slightly. This fluid also fills the open areas of the brain known as the ventricles. The brain is comprised of the:

Cortex	where most thinking functions occur
Cerebellum . .	which coordinates movement and balance
Brain Stem . .	which controls consciousness, alertness, and basic bodily functions such as breathing, respiration, and pulse.

The cortex is the largest part of the brain and is divided into two hemispheres. The dominant hemisphere (usually the left hemisphere) controls verbal functions (speaking, writing, reading, calculating), while the right hemisphere generally controls functions that are more visual-spatial in nature (visual memory, copying, drawing, rhythm). The illustration found on page 173 provides more specific information regarding the capacities of the left and right hemispheres of the brain.

Many characteristics are common among persons with injuries on the same side of the brain. Damage to the right side of the brain often results in impaired perceptions and paralysis on the left side of the body (i.e., left hemiplegia). Persons with injury to the left side of the brain manifest problems in communication related to speech, comprehension, reading, and writing, along with paralysis of the right side of the body. Persons with ABI often show changes in personality and emotional control no matter which side the injury occurred.

Left and Right Hemispheres of the Brain

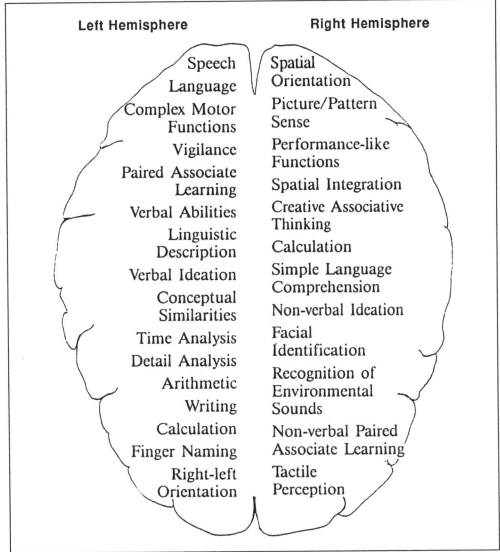

Left Hemisphere   **Right Hemisphere**

Left Hemisphere	Right Hemisphere
Speech	Spatial Orientation
Language	Picture/Pattern Sense
Complex Motor Functions	Performance-like Functions
Vigilance	Spatial Integration
Paired Associate Learning	Creative Associative Thinking
Verbal Abilities	Calculation
Linguistic Description	Simple Language Comprehension
Verbal Ideation	Non-verbal Ideation
Conceptual Similarities	Facial Identification
Time Analysis	Recognition of Environmental Sounds
Detail Analysis	Non-verbal Paired Associate Learning
Arithmetic	Tactile Perception
Writing	
Calculation	
Finger Naming	
Right-left Orientation	

The cortex can be further divided into four lobes, each of which specializes in particular functions and skills:

1. **Frontal Lobe** emotional control, motivation, social functioning, expressive language, inhibition of impulses, motor integration, voluntary movement.
2. **Temporal Lobe** memory, receptive, language, sequencing, musical awareness.
3. **Parietal Lobe** sensation, academic skills such as reading, awareness of spatial relationships.
4. **Occipital Lobe** visual perception.

Other complications that are secondary to head injury include:

1. Spasticity (hypertonic muscle, exaggerated stretch reflexes, flexion and extension synergies)
2. Connective tissue contractures
3. Bowel and bladder dysfunctions
4. Pneumonia
5. Epileptic seizures
6. Frozen Shoulder
7. Depression
8. Headaches

Most of the participants in post-secondary APE programs have incurred either a cerebrovascular accident or traumatic head injury. Although many of the clinical manifestations between these disabilities are similar, noticeable differences do exist, as illustrated in the following charts.

Differences Between Persons with Cerebrovascular Accident (CVA) and Acquired Brain Injury (ABI)

	CVA	HEAD TRAUMA
AGE	50+	16-25 (most common age)
INJURIES	Brain tissue and secondary dysfunctions	Brain, secondary dysfunctions orthopedic
BRAIN DAMAGE	Local, specific	General nonspecific
FAMILY	Head of household	Dependent or new head
VOCATION	Retirement or approaching	Unestablished, student
BEHAVIOR	Somewhat predictable	Unpredictable
SEXUALITY	Mature, adjusted	Immature, confused

Teaching Tips for Persons with Left and Right Hemiplegia

Left Brain Damage Right Hemiplegia	Tips
* Speech & Language Problems	* Speak slowly, use short sentences.

* Slow, Cautious & Disorganized
  Behavioral Styles
	* Give frequent and accurate
	  feedback.

* Memory Deficit Relating to Speech	* Be helpful but not a nag.

Right Brain Damage Left Hemiplegia	Tips

* Spatial-Perceptual Problems;
  i.e., decreased ability to judge
  distances, sizes, etc.
	* Have person demonstate
	  skills rather than taking
	  their word for it.

* Impulsive & Too Fast
  Behavioral Style
	* Have person talk self through
	  tasks.

* Over-Estimate Abilities	* Use caution.
* One-Sided Neglect	* Arrange environment to maximum sensory input.

Indicated Exercise Program

Often, individuals with ABI are resistant to physical activity on the basis that it will aggravate headaches, cause dizziness, or fatigue them. Generally, exercise will not aggravate any conditions. It is recommended that the individual spend at least 30 to 60 minutes daily participating in activities that will develop muscular strength and endurance, cardiovascular endurance, balance, and coordination. Small group activities teaching balance and range of motion have been found to be successful and beneficial, provided that progress is monitored regularly. The time spent partaking in exercise, swimming, and/or sports activities is not only valuable physically, but is also psychologically stimulating. Due to abnormal tone and reflexes typically associated with ABI, it is recommended that a physical therapist familiar with neurodevelopmental approaches provide input to the exercise program.

A suggested program for the participant with ABI should consist of the following:

Muscular Strength

Strength exercises are usually best performed using PNF or manual resistance. Which muscle groups to strengthen will depend upon which muscles are hypertonic and hypotonic. Typically, key muscle groups to strengthen include dorsiflexors, knee extensors and flexors, hip extensors and abductors, abdominals, wrist and finger extensors, and shoulder abductors. However, each person should be individually evaluated to determine specific needs. If using PNF, perform hold-relax prior to slow reversals to induce muscle relaxation. (Presently there is much discussion regarding weight training and CVA due to the fact that weight training may increase muscle tonus and inappropriate synergies).

Flexibility

Range of motion should be performed on all major joints - plantarflexors, hamstrings, hip flexors and adductors, and shoulder flexors and adductors. Contracture of the heel cord is typicaly and restricts the body moving over the ankle during stance phase of gait. When the ankle cannot dorsiflex in stance, the knee may hyperextend. Hold-relax techniques are preferable to active or passive ROM.

Balance and Coordination

For some persons with ABI, a significant portion of the exercise program will be devoted to balance activities and coordination. Loss of equilibrium reactions and the re-emergence of primitive reflexes limit the repertoire of gross motor activities, including ambulation. The balance exercises presented in Chapter 10 are ideally suited for persons with ABI and promote the achievement of standing and walking. If a participant is unable to sit independently because of extensor hypertonicity, the tone can be reduced by rotating and flexing the trunk at the hips (Umphred, 1985). Abduction and external rotation of the upper extremities further normalizes tone.

Gross motor activities need to interesting, goal-directed, and functional; for example, dribbling or kicking a ball, throwing and catching, jumping rope, and dancing. Many activities can be obtained from developmental charts.

Cardiovascular Training

This activity is not only useful to increase aerobic capacity, but calms an agitated participant, and encourages reciprocal movements of the legs in preparation for ambulation. Endurance should be addressed because low fitness levels may interfere with daily rigors of rehabilitation. Obtain medical clearance prior to allowing a participant with a stroke to engage in a cardiovascular program.

Perceptual-Motor

Many head injuries display deficiencies with spatial awareness (ability to judge time, distance, sizes, etc.), right/left discrimination, atopographic memory loss, etc. Many of the activities listed in Chapter 10 are appropriate.

Communicating with a Person with Aphasia

Many times the person with ABI will suffer from aphasia, the inability to comprehend spoken language (receptive aphasia) and/or execute speech (expressive aphasia). These deficits are due to damage in the auditory cortex of the brain. The following list contains suggestions for communicating with persons with aphasia.

1. Allow the person to make mistakes while speaking. Occasional corrections are appropriate. If corrected too often, the person may not want to speak.
2. Do not interrupt the person or supply words unless help is requested.
3. Some responses may be unrelated to what the person actually wants to say. Casually restating what was said may help the person in correcting errors.
4. Don't force the person to speak to people when he/she doesn't want to.
5. Don't speak for the person unless asked or absolutely necessary.
6. The person with aphasia often has to stop after a few words to think of the next word. Don't supply the word at this point.
7. Don't be overly optimistic with the person in regard to regaining speech (i.e., do not suggest that speech will return soon).
8. Build up the person's confidence by emphasizing the activities he/she can do.
9. Encourage the aphasic in all of his/her efforts. Raise even the smallest gain.
10. Don't take it for granted that the person with aphasia understands what you are saying. Occasionally have the person repeat what is expected of him/her.
11. Keep material short, simple and concrete. Give directions in short phrases, rather than single words of long sentences.
12. Reword what you've said in various ways if the person doesn't understand the first time.
13. The person with aphasia is an adult. Treat him/her like one.

Amputations

Definition

Amputation refers to the loss of an upper or lower extremity. The term includes both acquired and congenital limb losses.

Etiology

1. Trauma (where reconstructive surgery was not feasible)
2. Peripheral Vascular Disease
3. Diabetes
4. Frostbite
5. Chronic Infection of Bone (e.g., osteomyelitis)
6. Tumor
7. Congenital Deformity where existing limb was not capable of functioning properly.

The "phantom limb" syndrome is a frequent complaint of the person with a amputation. This syndrome refers to the persistent awareness of the removed limb. This pain may occur shortly after surgery or later. Generally, these sensations are temporary, becoming less common once the prosthesis is applied.

Types of Amputations
(according to the site and level of loss)

Congenital Absences (birth defects)	Amputation Level
Amelia (terminal transverse)	Shoulder Disarticulation
Hemimelia (terminal transverse)	Above the Elbow (AE)
Partial Hemimelia	Below the Elbow (BE)
Acheiria	Wrist Disarticulation; Trans-metacarpal Amputation
Amelia (terminal transverse)	Hip Disarticulation
Hemimelia (terminal transverse)	Above the Knee (AK)
Partial Hemimelia	Below the Knee (BK)
Apodi	Syme Amputation
Adactylia.	Trans-metatarsal Amputation

Hemimelia denotes one-half of a limb. Amelia refers to total absence of a limb.

Inidcated Exercise Program

The initial rehabilitation program for a person with an amputation consists of training in the use of the prosthesis. For the person with a lower extremity amputation this includes:

1. Balance activities
2. Ambulation
3. Pivoting
4. Stair climbing
5. How to fall to and rise from the ground

After this stage, the exercise treatment should develop strength and endurance in both the impaired and normal extremities. Manual resistance would be employed for strengthening the stump.

The aerobic capacity of the person should be maintained as much as possible. Swimming is an excellent aerobic choice for even the person with a bilateral BK. Swim fins may be attached to the stumps by special prosthesis. Arm crank ergometry may be another choice for those with limited weight-bearing capabilities. Some persons may use the leg cycle ergometer while wearing their prostheses.

Arthritis

Definition

Arthritis literally means inflammation of a joint. The definition is a little misleading as many types of arthritis do not evidence joint inflammation. Arthritis is used to describe nearly 100 different conditions which cause aches and pain in the joint or surrounding connective tissue. Several of the most common forms are osteoarthritis, rheumatoid arthritis, anklyosing spondylitis, and gout. Children are affected by certain types of arthritis as well as adults.

Osteoarthritis is a degenerative condition usually associated with aging, although it can occur in young people. It affects the cartilage of the joints and is localized, particularly in the weight-bearing areas (i.e., spine, hips, knees, and ankles). Degenerative wear and tear of the articulating surface of a joint is characteristic of this condition. Inflammation can be, but is usually not present. Most people over 65 years of age are affected by OA to some degree. Injury or consistent strain can also lead to OA. The diagnosis of osteoarthritis is usually based upon an x-ray coupled with blood tests. The prognosis is usually good as the condition progresses slowly, even in severe cases. Profound crippling is relatively rare. Degenerative wear and tear of the articulating surface of a joint is characteristic of this condition. Inflammation can be, but is usually not present. Most people over 65 years of age are affected by OA to some degree. Injury or consistent strain can also lead to OA.

Unlike osteoarthritis, **rheumatoid arthritis** often begins before the age of 40 years and is inflammatory. It is typical to see periods of inflammation (i.e., exacerbations) followed by remissions. The time interval of exacerbations and remissions will vary among individuals. The site of inflammation is the synovial membrane. Normally, the synovial membrane contributes to the production of synovial fluid (which nourishes joint cartilage and keeps the joint lubricated) and provides for removal of synovial fluid from the joint. Inflammation of the synovial lining results in impairment of both functions. An excess of joint fluid is produced, the drainage mechanism becomes inadequate, and fluid becomes trapped within the capsule. This process damages the capsule, ligaments, cartilage, and bone. This mechanical stress makes the joint vulnerable to overstretching during functional use. Pain results due to the increased intra-articular pressure on the innervated capsule. Symptoms of inflammation include pain, swelling, warmth, and decreased range of motion. In rheumatoid arthritis, inflammation usually symmetrically affects the smaller joints (i.e., hands, elbows, feet). It is systemic, causing generalized fatigue, decreased appetite, and weight loss. Symptoms of an exacerbation include loss of appetite, fatigue, fever, and the development of rheumatoid nodules which form under the skin. Various blood tests help the physician recognize rheumatoid arthritis. X-rays are not very useful in diagnosis because it takes several months before the changes in the bones and cartilage appear. It is estimated that only one in six people with rheumatoid arthritis develop any deformities. Rheumatiod arthritis can affect people of any age, including children (juvenile rheumatoid arthritis) and there is a greater incidence in women.

Ankylosing spondylitis is a chronic form of arthritis which occurs primarily in individuals under 35 years. The etiology of the disease is unknown. However, many individuals have a genetic marker known as B-27. Generally, ankylosing spondylitis begins with pain and stiffness in the lower back and progresses up the spine. It may eventually involve the hips, shoulders, and occasionally the knees. Although the symptoms may disappear spontaneously, the extent of rigidity that has occurred will remain.

Gouty arthritis is caused by an inherited metabolic disorder which allows uric acid to accumulate in the blood. Crystals of uric acid are then deposited in the joints, promoting inflammation. The most common site of deposition is the big toe, but other joints may be affected. Gout is an extremely painful condition as the joint becomes hot, red and swollen.

Indicated Exercise Program

Unfortunately, many people with arthritis think exercise is harmful. Others become discouraged because progress is slow or their exercises are painful. Participation in specially designed exercise programs can significantly contribute to decreased pain and increased functional level. Range of motion exercises will increase joint mobility and lubrication, strengthening exercises will increase stability of vulnerable joints, and endurance exercises will promote cardiovascular fitness. Programs must be designed to meet the needs for each person. It is critically important that individuals with arthritis increase their understanding of the disease so that they may use good judgement regarding necessary exercise modifications.

Research to determine appropriate exercise programs has been difficult due to the spontaneous course of exacerbations and remissions. Arthritis also affects people in different parts of their bodies and to varying degrees — everyone is unique. For the participant with rheumatoid arthritis, careful consideration must be given to the proper combination of rest and exercise. Rest is necessary to reduce inflammation; yet, disuse also allows the joints to become stiff and the muscles to atrophy. As a general rule, the intensity and duration of exercise should be determined by pain.

Along with drug therapy, surgery, and good health habits, regular range of motion is the indicated treatment for most forms of arthritis. All major joints should be gently placed through their range of motion several times daily. Active stretching of joints is preferable to passive because it aids in maintaining the strength of muscle groups that oppose a contracture. Flexibility exercises should always be performed through the pain-free range of motion.

It is paramount to keep the body weight under control. Obesity accelerates the damage to diseased, weight-bearing joints. Aerobic exercises such as swimming and bicycling at low resistances are recommended over jogging. Many hospitals have instituted "arthroswim" programs for their outpatients with arthritis.

Strength exercises are indicated if they are performed actively, isometrically, or with gentle resistance. PNF is especially beneficial as it strengthens all muscles about a joint. Traction and approximation should not be performed when utilizing PNF techniques. Key muscle groups to strengthen generally include the extensors of the hip, knee, fingers, wrist, and elbow.

Contraindications

1. Avoid exercising with the presence of pain other than the discomfort from normal exercise exertion.
2. Use of isotonic weight equipment for strength training causes excessive compression of joints or traction-loading.
3. Do not perform neck hyperextensions or pushups with the hands.

When Should Exercise be Performed?

1. On a daily basis.
2. When there is the least amount of pain and stiffness during the day.
3. When the individual is least tired.
4. When the individual receives the maximum benefit from medications during the day (generally 10-11 am).
5. After preparation with massage, heating pad, warm shower, or gentle rhythmic movements.

Precautions

1. Find out what type of arthritis the participant has.
2. Minimize stress to joints. Teach about selection of appropriate activities such as swimming.
3. Avoid vigorously exercising an inflamed joint, but gently put joint through range of motion.
4. Discourage increasing medications without physician's approval.
5. Wear warm clothes.
6. Modify the exercise routine with how the person feels. The arthritic condition will fluctuate from worse to better on a daily basis.
7. Use the two-hour rule: If exercise-induced pain lasts longer than two hours, then cut back on intensity, but do not stop exercising altogether (e.g., decrease repetitions or force).
8. Individualize the exercise program to address problem areas.

Description Arthroswim Program
("Arthroswim" — Arthritis Foundation, San Diego Area Chapter)

The Arthroswim Program deals with a diverse group of participants whose expression of disease is wide and varied. Therefore, the program must also be wide and varied to meet their needs.

Explanation to Instructors

This exercise program has essentially been divided into five parts:

1. Warm Up Exercise
2. Stretching Exercise
3. Aerobic Cardiopulmonary Exercise
4. Strengthening Exercise
5. Cool Down Exercise

A new swimmer (a student not now actively swimming at least twice a week for approximately 20 minutes) may find it to be less painful and most beneficial to do the warm up and stretching portions on the first visit to class. Then, as the student continues to attend, the aerobic exercise and then lastly (approximately the third visit to class) the strengthening exercises and cool down activities may be added **slowly**. This approach allows some program flexibility to be applied individually to each student as per the student's needs.

The previous paragraph may also be applied to students returning from vacation/ hospital stay/illness/arthritis flare-up.

Students should be encouraged to **always** consult their physician about changes in anything having to do with their arthritis (i.e., medications, pain, endurance, strength, complications from a fall, accident, fever, etc.).

Class Variables:

1. Repetitions
2. Speed of pulling an arm/leg through the water
3. Walk-Jog-Run
4. Time spent in water
5. Duration of each exercise
6. Rest periods
7. Water depth-buoyancy
8. Fun
9. Type of arthritis
10. Stationary exercise (standing still for each exercise — walking forward and backward with water resistance — not a variable)

Arthroswim Program

Introduction

Every person in the class must be considered individually. All exercises are not for everyone. The best rule is: If it hurts, STOP!

Warm-Up

Strengthening Exercises

1. **Pelvic Tilt:** Place back against the wall with knees slightly bent, push the small of your back and shoulders flat against the wall, hold this position and do some breathing exercise like counting or singing.
2. **Shoulder Girdle Rolling:** With arms at side, roll shoulders in a circle (forwards and backwards).
3. **Single Knee to Chest:** Take three steps and pull one bent knee to your chest, alternating knees.
4. **Shoulder External Rotation:** Elbows bent with fingertips toward shoulders, squeeze elbows to touching in front of your jaw, stretch elbows out to the side and breathe deeply.
5. **Isometric Knee Exercise:** With low back flat against the wall, tighten ankles to lift toes and tighten knees very straight, hold and relax toes and knees.

6. **Shoulder Internal Rotation**: With hands behind your back, bend elbows to reach towards shoulder blades, breathe in deeply, relax and exhale as you lower hands.
7. **Neck Exercise**: Pull head back keeping chin level as if at attention, lower shoulders and inhale deeply, relax neck and shoulders as you exhale.
8. **Heel Cord Stretching**: Face wall placing forearms against the wall standing with one foot in front of the other, keeping heels on floor, bend front knee and slowly lean toward wall until a pull is felt at heel of back leg. Push out with arms to standing position.
9. **Pronation and Supination**: With elbows at rib cage and palms facing down, push palms down through the water until elbows are straight, now turn palms up and pull up through the water keeping elbows at rib cage.
10. **Finger Curls**: Squeeze hands into a fist, uncurl so that fingertips touch the base of fingers, then stretch fingers and thumbs out very straight. Repeat, curl, fist, uncurl and stretch.

Running, Cardiopulmonary Activity, Swimming Laps, Walking, Hopping

Work Out

1. **Hula**: Rotate hips around in a large circle.
2. **Around the World**: With side to the wall, bend outside knee to chest, stretch leg out to side, touch foot to floor, then stretch leg behind you.
3. **Sweep and Pull**: Sweep one hand to opposite shoulder and pull away to straighten elbow, alternate.
4. **Pendulum**: With low back flat against wall, raise one leg out to the side, drop leg to touch floor and stretch across body to opposite side, swing leg down to touch floor and raise leg out to the side again. Repeat, then swing other leg.
5. **Squeeze and Stretch**: Squeeze hands reaching out in front of body, stretch hands open and press straight arms close to body and back behind body, bring arms forward without turning hands.
6. **Can-Can**: Pull one knee to chest, kick foot and lower leg in and out.
7. **Breast-stroke Arms**: While walking across pool, do breast-stroke with palms down.
8. **Leg Circles**: With side to wall, raise outside leg and circle leg forwards and backwards.
9. **Pull and Leap**: Starting position — arms out to side walking sideways, pull hands and arms up and out to chest height.
10. **Ankle Exercise**: Pull one knee to chest, point foot up and down several times, then circle foot in both directions.
11. **Radial Strengthening**: With elbows touching rib cage and palms facing each other, tilt hands to thumb side, pointing thumb and fingers towards ceiling, hold and then relax hands back to beginning position.
12. **Heel and Toe**: Walk up on toes for three steps, then walk on heels for three steps.

Cool Down

Asthma

Definition

Asthma is classified as a reversible (spontaneous or therapeutically) obstructive airway disease, resulting in the sudden onset of muscle spasms, swelling, and the presence of mucous in the tracheobronchial tree. It is caused by a hyperirritability to a variety of stimuli (inhalants, ingestants, environment, exercise). Exercise-induced asthma (EIA) is brought on by sustained exercise such as running or bicycling for longer than 6 minutes.

Symptoms

1. Cough or hack (due to increased mucous)
2. Wheezing and dyspnea, leading to difficult exhalation
3. Severe bronchial constriction where individual becomes cyanotic, constituting an extreme medical emergency

Emergency Procedures for Asthma Attack

1. Have individual sit and attempt to relax.
2. Provide glass of warm water to break-down mucous.
3. Administer medication.

The following information should be in the participant's medical file:

1. Type and frequency of medication.
2. Possible side effects of drugs.
3. Procedures to follow during an attack.
4. Substances which trigger the attack (allergies).
5. Anecdotal record of all attacks.

Physical Characteristics of Persons with Asthma

1. Weak abdominals.
2. Loss of flexibility in the shoulder, low back, and hamstrings.
3. Weak upper back muscles (rhomboids).
4. Reduced FEV_1 during and after cessation of exercise. FEV_1 refers to the forced expiratory volume of air in one second. It is a flow rate measuring the amount of air (liters) expired in one second from a maximal exhalation. It is usually expressed as a percentage of the total amount of exhaled air (Forced Vital Capacity or FVC). In unaffected subjects, 80% of the FVC should be expired within the first second. During sustained exercise, FEV_1 falls below 60% in persons with asthma. A drop in FEV_1 below 80% is one parameter signaling the onset of asthma. EIA becomes increasingly severe as the duration of exercise is increased. The response appears to be greatest after 6 to 8 minutes of aerobic activity.

Indicated Exercise Program

The following outline provides recommended activities to help prevent the onset of EIA:

Warm Up (Sufficient duration to break a sweat.)

It appears that bronchoconstrictors are slowly depleted during warm up.

1. Walking alternated with slow jog (equal periods of walk and jog).
2. Strengthening activities for the abdominals and upper back.
3. Rhythmic and gentle calisthenics.
4. Interval or anaerobic activity.

Main Activity

1. Swimming. Found to be one aerobic activity which is not asthmogenic (asthma-provoking).
2. Team sports/anaerobic activities: Volleyball, softball, tennis, etc.
3. If jogging or cycling program is instituted, begin with intervals (three bouts of three minutes with rest periods). Increase duration as tolerated.

Warm Down

1. Flexibility exercises for shoulders, low back, hamstrings, hip flexors, and ankles.
2. Should be a low level activity for 5 minutes or until heart rate returns to within 20 beats per minute of resting level.

Cerebral Palsy

Definition

Cerebral palsy is a non-progressive disorder of movement and posture appearing early in life (before 5 years) and resulting from insult to the immature brain. The lesion is permanent but presents no further degeneration. There exist several distinct types, depending upon the site of the lesion.

Etiology

1. Birth Trauma (cerebral hemorrhage) — insufficient oxygen
2. Prematurity
3. Rubella
4. Rh factor
5. Child Abuse

Types of Cerebral Palsy

Spastic

1. Hyperactive tonic and phasic stretch reflexes (hypertonic muscle and exaggerated tendon reflexes, respectively)
2. Clonus (reverberating jerky movements).
3. Lesion to motor cortex.
4. Postural deformities secondary to spasticity and contractures (e.g., spastic crouch, scoliosis).
5. Scissors gait — excessive hip flexion-adduction-internal rotation, knee flexion, plantarflexion.

Athetoid

1. Rotary and dystonic movements (distorted positions).
2. Range of motion is normal.
3. Lesion to basal ganglia.

Ataxic

1. Disturbance of balance.
2. Hypotonic muscle tone.
3. Lesion to cerebellum.

Associated Characteristics (not present in all individuals)

1. Seizures
2. Mental retardation
3. Impairment of sight, hearing, and speech
4. Perceptual problems and learning disabilities
5. Motor deficits
6. Strabismus

Indicated Exercise Program for Spastic Cerebral Palsy

Restore Muscular Balance at All Affected Joints

1. Resistive exercises for atrophied and lengthened muscle. This typically includes: hip extensors, abductors, and external rotators; knee extensors; dorsiflexors; elbow, wrist, and finger extensors.
2. Provide range of motion for hip flexors, hip adductors, knee flexors, plantarflexors, wrist flexors, elbow flexors, shoulders. Use hold-relax or active stretching techniques if possible. Passive stretching often has to be instituted for persons more severely involved (see Chapter 7).

Indicated Exercise Program for All Types of Cerebral Palsy

1. Increase cardiovascular endurance through arm or leg cycling, swimming, running, or wheelchair pushing.
2. Balance activities for lying, kneeling, sitting, and standing position (see Chapter 10).
3. Perceptual motor activities, especially manipulative activities involving grasp and release.
4. Activities promoting control of reciprocal movement: Climbing, skipping, marching, cycling, stepping in and out of tires, and swimming.
5. Practice walking, concentrating on heelstrike.
6. Kinetron for strength and endurance.
7. Careful positioning of and hand placement on the person with cerebral palsy will prevent the avtivation of abnormal tone. For example, in ambulatory persons with athetoid cerebral palsy, spontaneous depression or elevation of a scapula or protraction of a shoulder will often induce tone changes throughout the body (Umphred, 1985). If the initiating action can be inhibited, while righting reactions of the head and trunk are facilitated, more normal tone and movement are presented. Visual, auditory, and emotional stimuli may also trigger unwanted tone and posture. Physical therapists can provide suggestions for proper positioning and handling of a person with cerebral palsy.

Diabetes

Diabetes is a disease in which the body is unable to use food properly. It is caused by an insufficient supply of insulin which is normally produced in the pancreas. The function of insulin is to regulate the rate at which the body uses or stores sugar. Much of the food we eat is converted into a form of sugar called glucose or stored as glycogen. Glycogen is stored in the liver and muscles and may be broken down into glucose when needed. Insulin is needed by the body to burn glucose which provides energy for the muscles. If the pancreas fails to produce enough insulin, glucose cannot be used by the muscles or stored and accumulates in the bloodstream, causeing blood sugar levels to rise above normal.

Two signs of diabetes are: (1) excessive amounts of sugar in the blood (hyperglycemia) and (2) excretion of sugar in the urine (glycosuria). The symptoms of diabetes are related to the increased amount of sugar in the blood. Diabetes may be without symptoms - such may be the case with elderly persons. In adults, common symptoms are sweating, palpitation, tremor, and weakness. Other symptoms include pain, numbness, tingling in the hands and feet, disturbances in vision, irritability, and nervousness. In children, classic symptoms such as weight loss, polyuria, polydipsia, and fatigue are manifested.

There are two types of diabetes:

1. Juvenile diabetes, insulin-dependent
2. Adult onset diabetes, non-insulin dependent.

Juvenile diabetes generally begins in adolescence and can develop rapidly with acute symptoms. Adult onset diabetes is less abrupt and results in resistance to the individual's own insulin. However, both types may occur at any age.

Diabetes can lead to:

1. **Cardiovascular Disorders.** A person with diabetes is two times more likely to develop Coronary Artery Disease.
2. **Macrovascular Disease.** Diabetes contributes to the development of Peripheral Vascular Disease, sometimes resulting in amputation.
3. **Microvascular Disease.** Diabetic retinopathy results when tiny blood vessels in the retina break and cause little hemorrhages on or near the retina. This can lead to permanent visual loss (blindness) over time. Cataracts also seem to be more prevalent in persons with diabetes. Because of the relationship between diabetes and eye disorders, the diabetic should always inform an ophthalmologist about his/her condition.
4. **Sensorimotor and Autonomic Neuropathy.** Destruction of sensory, motor, and autonomic nerves caused by excessive blood glucose and poor blood supply.
5. **Renal Nephropathy.** Renal dysfunction.

Treatment

Diabetes cannot be cured, but can be controlled. Treatment may include medication (insulin), daily exercise, and diet therapy. Exercise in consistent amounts is very important in managing Type 2 diabetes. Blood glucose levels should be checked prior to exercise to determine any adjustments in food intake. If blood sugar levels are 300 mg or greater, **do not begin exercise**. In this case, metabolic control of glucose will become even more dysfunctional. The following chart provides guidelines for adjusting food intake according to blood sugar levels.

Guidelines for Adjusting Food Intake According to Blood Sugar Levels

Type of Exercise and Examples	If Blood Sugar Is	Increase Food Intake By	Suggested Foods
Exercise of short duration and of low to moderate intensity	Less than 100 mg	10-15 gms of carbohydrate per hour	1 fruit or 1 bread exchange
Examples: Walking a 1/2 mile or leisurely bicycling for 30 minutes.	100 mg or above	Not necessary to increase food	
Exercise of moderate intensity	Less than 100 mg	25-50 gms of carbohydrate before exercise, then 10-15 gms per hour of exercise	1/2 meat sandwich with a milk or fruit exchange
Examples: Tennis, swimming, jogging, leisurely bicycling, gardening, golfing, or vacuuming for one hour	100-200 mg	10-15 gms of carbohydrate per hour of exercise	1 fruit or 1 bread exchange
	200-300 mg	Not necessary to increase food	
	300 mg or greater	Don't begin exercise until blood glucose is under control	
Strenuous activity or exercise	Less than 100 mg	50 gms of carbohydrate, monitor blood glucose carefully	1 meat sandwich (2 slices of bread) with a milk and fruit exchange
Examples: Football, hockey, racquetball or basketball games; strenuous biking or swimming, and shoveling heavy snow for one hour	100-170 mg	25-50 mg of carbohydrate, depending on intensity and duration	1/2 meat sandwich with a mik or fruit exchange
	200-300 mg	10-15 gms of carbohydrate per hour of exercise	1 fruit or 1 bread exchange

Diabetic Reactions and Treatment

The acute complications of diabetes are insulin reaction and diabetic coma. The former will most likely occur during an exercise session because the effects of exercise and insulin are similar except where blood sugar levels exceed 300 mg. If the levels of blood glucose are insufficient to fuel the brain, then symptoms appear, such as confusion, nausea and blurred vision. Administering fruit juices, non-dietetic carbonated beverages, or hard candies usually will terminate the insulin reaction in two to three minutes. If the person with diabetes does not respond promptly to sugar, medical help should be sought immediately. (Bleck, 1975).

The Effects of Too Much or Too Little Insulin

	Insulin Reaction	Diabetic Coma
Onset:	Rapid (minutes)	Gradual (hours)
Symptoms:	Headache Nausea Vomiting Tremulousness Irritability	Fatigue Thirst Hunger Frequent Urination
Skin:	Cold and Moist	Warm and Dry
Breathing:	Normal and Shallow	Deep
Urine:	Negative Glucose Negative Acetone	4+ Glucose Positive Acetone
Treatment:	Sugar	Insulin Medical Attention

Indicated Exercise Program

All persons with diabetes should undergo a medical evaluation and exercise assessment prior to participation in an exercise program to rule out occult cardiovascular disease and manifestations of secondary diabetic complications. The mode of exercise and type of prescription will depend on what type of diabetic complications the participant has. The reader is referred to an indepth discussion of appropriate exercises and safety concerns for persons with diabetic complications by Graham and Lasko-McCarthey (1990).

In general, aerobic exercise is the recommendation for most persons with diabetes as it improves cardiovascular function, lipid profiles, weight control, and insulin sensitivity. Jogging, swimming, cycling, and low-impact aerobics are examples of aerobic activities that can be performed at 65-80% of maximal heart rate for at least 30 minutes, three to four times per week. Because of the high incidence of silent cardiovascular disease, caution needs to be used when prescribing exercise intensity — untrained, older individuals need to begin at a lower intensity. Include proper warm-up and cooldown.

High-intensity exercises involve anaerobic metabolism and do not elicit the same benefits as aerobic exercise. For the person without diabetic complications, high-intensity exercise such as weight training is usually safe. However, for the person with diabetes-related vascular disease, this type of exercise is potentially harmful and should be avoided - due to the hemodynamic process that occurs in Valsalva-type maneuvers and results in elevated systolic blood pressure and potential hemorrhage in the eye.

Exercise with Peripheral Vascular Disease (PVD). Interval training (e.g., alternate 2-min walks with 1-min rests), swimming, stationary cycling, walking on a slow treadmill at 1 mph, and chair exericses are all options for persons with PVD. Chair exercises or upper body exercises can be performed by those who are unable to use the lower extremities due to PVD and claudication; recumbent and non-weight-bearing activities are good choices. A clinical recommendation during aerobic activity is for the participant to establish an exercise intensity that is balanced between his/her target heart rate and Grade II pain (moderate discomfort or pain from which the person's attention can be diverted by a number of stimuli such as conversation; American College of Sports Medicine, 1986). For example, if a participant cannot achieve the minimum target heart rate because it elicits pain above Grade II, then lower the target heart rate until a Grade II pain is achieved. Precaution - discontinue any exercise provokes pain at Grade III (intense pain from which the person's cannot be diverted except by catastrophic events) or above.

Exercise with Diabetic Retinopathy. Aerobic exercise for persons with retinopathy includes stationary cycling, low-intensity rowing on a rowing machine, swimming, walking, and jogging. Adaptations for accomplishing these activities can be found under "Visual Impairments" at the end of this chapter. Greenlee (1987) recommended that the heart rate not exceed that which elicits a systolic blood pressure of 170 mm Hg. The blood pressure should be monitored during every exercise session and intensity adjusted accordingly. This method is used because moderate exercise can raise systolic blood pressure to levels above 200 mm Hg, risking furhter damage to the retina. A submaximal pretest should be conducted to establish initial exercise intensity. Resistive exercise using standard weight-lifting equipment is not recommended (unless a person is totally blind); however, if a weight-lifting regime is strongly desired by the participant, physician approval is requisite. For each resistive exercise, the load to be lifted should be such that the person can lift a minimum of 15 repetitions per set with a resistance that does not cause undue fatigue. Exhaling on the lift/effort and inhaling on the return to starting position will prevent a Valsalva maneuver. For additional exercise recommendations for persons with retinopathy, see the section on "Visual Impairments" later in this chapter.

At present there is no clear evidence that intensive physical training programs accelerate the progression of diabetic retinopathy. However, certain types of exercise result in large increases of systolic blood pressure with concomitant increases in intraocular pressure; these exercises are contraindicated. Specifically, activities should be avoided that involve (1) bending over so that the head is positioned lower than the waist, (2) Valsalva-type maneuvers that raise blood pressure, (3) any near maximal isometric contractions, (4) weight lifting with high resistance and low repetitions, (5) vigorous bouncing such as high impact aerobics, (6) rapid eye-head movements found in contact sports, and (7) strenuous upper extremity exercise such as rowing and arm cycle ergometry (Graham & Lasko-McCarthey, 1990). The breath should never be held during an exercise effort. Strenuous upper extremity exercise increases peripheral resistance to blood flow, resulting in higher blood pressure. Jogging can produce irregular head movements that may potentially aggravate an eye condition. Additional activities that are contraindicated include parachuting, scuba diving, and yoga. The latter uses postures which increase intraocular pressure. Exercise is contraindicated if the person has recently undergone retinal photocoagulation treatment or eye surgery.

Exercise with Renal Nephropathy. Because of the many complications of diabetes and renal disease, thorough screening prior to initiation of an exercise progam is essential. No exercise program should begin until the person is stabilized on a therapeutic program of medication, dialysis, and diet. Persons on hemodialysis benefit from aerobic exercise such as brisk walking, cycling, and swimming. The program should begin gradually due to anemia, cardiovascular dysfunction, and low physical work capacity, using an interval training (5 min work, 5 min rest). Intensity of exercise should range from 60-80% of the person's maximum heart rate. Fluid replacement is warranted if exercise is performed in heat or following dialysis treatment.

Exercise with Sensorimotor Neuropathy. Persons with this type of neuropathy are more dependent on vision when performing motor skills because proprioception is diminished in the extremities.

The list below provides strategies to facilitate movement in persons with sensorimotor neuropathy (Graham & Lasko-McCarthey, 1990):

1. Use mirrors to facilitate body awareness of the lower extremities.
2. Enhance muscle tone by rubbing and tapping the dermatome (skin) of the muscle to be contracted.
3. Use visual aids such as footprints placed on the floor during gait training.
4. Teach principles of equilibrium such as (a) hands out to side, (b) lowering the center of gravity by bending knees, and (c) focusing on stationary object at eye level.
5. Increase proprioception and stimulate joint reflexes adding resistance to the movement (e.g., wrist weights or manually applied resistance).
6. Use non-weight bearing activities such as arm exercises, swimming, and cycling for persons with loss of sensation to the feet.
7. Inspect the feet before and after exercising for swelling, heat, redness, or ulcerations. Change shoes every 5 hours.
8. Use towels or canes to facilitate stretching exercises.
9. Use external support such as a chair during balance exercises.

Exercises with Autonomic Neuropathy. Stationary cycling or water exercises are suggested; the latter is particularly beneficial for persons with orthostatic hypertension because pressure of the water surrounding the body helps to maintain normal blood pressure. Sitting or semirecumbent (which assists in maintaining blood pressure) exercises are also recommended for developing fitness levels. Strenuous exercise involving rapid changes in body position should be avoided as the concomitant changes in heart rate and blood pressure may trigger a hypotensive episode following exercise.

Epilepsy

Definition

Epilepsy is symptomatic of a central nervous system disorder and results in excessive electrical discharges in the cerebrum (i.e., seizure). Epilepsy is a syndrome in which seizures occur repeatedly and is classified according to the severity of electrical discharge and the brain region where it originates.

Diagnosis

Diagnosis of epilepsy involves a complete physical and neurological examination and occasionally a spinal tap. The electroencephalogram (EEG) is useful, not only in identifying epilepsy, but determining the most effective treatment. This method records the brain's electrical patterns on a graph.

Etiology

1. Idiopathic (cause unknown)
2. Genetic disposition (possible metabolic disorder)
3. Acquired (tumors, anoxic brain, hemorrhage)
4. Prenatal (infections, rubella)
5. Postnatal (infections such as meningitis)

Factors Which Provoke Onset of a Seizure

1. Increased alkalinity of blood (dietary fat and exercise will increase acidity of blood)
2. Flashing strobe lights
3. Emotional stress
4. Edema
5. Hyperventilation at rest
6. Excessive fatigue

Types of Epilepsy

Absence (Petit Mal)

This type is more common in children than adults and frequently disappears in adolescence. It is a very mild form of seizure. Although the individual is unconscious during the seizure (5-20 seconds), the posture is maintained and convulsions do not occur. The only signs may be staring with rapid blinking or rolling of the eyes upward. Absence seizures may occur up to 100 times per day.

Tonic-Clonic (Grand Mal)

The tonic-clonic seizure has two phases which last a total of approximately five minutes. In the tonic phase, the individual becomes unconscious and rigid, falling to the ground. The clonic phase follows, characterized by rhythmic, muscular convulsions. After the seizure has ceased, the individual is very tired and may need to rest or sleep. These seizures often occur during sleep.

Complex-Partial (Psychomotor)

This type of seizure involves only a portion of the brain and presents varying symptoms among individuals, depending upon the portion of the brain affected. The duration of the seizure is usually between two to five minutes. The person often will perform purposeless, repetitive movements such as picking at clothing or rubbing of the hands. It is not unusual for the individual to walk around and he/she should be steered clear of any danger.

Any type of seizure may be preceded by an aura. This is an unusual feeling or sensation such as disturbed vision or a peculiar taste in the mouth. Seizures are characteristic and prevalent in persons with suspected brain damage such as cerebral palsy, mental retardation, learning disabilities, autism, and traumatic head injuries.

Indicated Exercise Program

Historically, vigorous physical education and competitive/contact sports were contraindicated by physicians for persons with epilepsy. It was assumed that additional head trauma from contact during sports might increase the incidence or intensity of seizures. However, research studies have never substantiated this notion. Furthermore, since aerobic exercise actually increases the acidity of the blood (due to metabolic acidosis), moderate physical activity may actually create a "buffer" against tonic-clonic seizures. The adapted physical educator should be cautioned, however, that over-fatigue may be a factor in all types of seizures, especially complex-partial (psychomotor) epilepsy.

When selecting physical activities, consider the individual's desire to participate and weigh it against medical management of the condition. Well-controlled seizures usually indicate unrestricted participation in contact sports, swimming, and tumbling. ALWAYS OBTAIN A MEDICAL CLEARANCE FROM A PHYSICIAN BEFORE ALLOWING THE INDIVIDUAL TO PARTICIPATE IN AN EXERCISE PROGRAM. Close supervision is always a must, especially in any activity involving heights or a pool.

First Aid for a Tonic-Clonic (Grand Mal) Epileptic Seizure

1. Keep calm. The person is usually not suffering or in danger.
2. Help person to a safe place, but DO NOT restrain convulsions.
3. Loosen tight clothing and protect his/her head from injury by placing something soft underneath it. If the person is wearing a helmet with straps (or any type of head gear with straps), remove it completely.

4. As soon as possible, turn the person on his/her side. This position will prevent the tongue from falling to the back of the throat and blocking the air passage. Choking from vomit or saliva will also be prevented by having the person on his/her side.
5. DO NOT PUT ANYTHING BETWEEN THE TEETH.
6. DO NOT give him/her anything to drink.
7. Stand by until the person has fully recovered consciousness and from the confusion which sometimes follows a seizure.
8. Let him/her rest if tired.
9. It is rarely necessary to call public authorities, a doctor, or an ambulance. However, in cases of repeated or prolonged seizures (over 10 minutes of stiffening or jerking), it is suggested that medical help be secured.
10. Fill out an anecdotal record provided by the instructor (see Appendix F). It is important to observe the progression of the seizure, especially if it is a first-time occurrence. The diagnosis of the type of seizure can be greatly aided by your observations. Inform the participant that an anecdotal record was written up on the seizure.
11. If injured, it may be necessary to call the paramedics. Fill out an injury report form.

Gerontology

Aging is a progressive, irreversible, and cumulative series of structural and functional changes that occur throughout one's life. Studies show that cells are lost from many tissues during the process of aging. Organs gradually change their structure and function less efficiently in older individuals.

Particularly frightening is the loss of physical and mental abilities associated with aging. Physical fitness enhances both the mental and physical health of older persons. The purpose of exercise is not to add years to one's life, but rather add life to one's years!

Degeneration associated with aging should be distinguished from disease and disuse. Aging is often associated with weight gain, an accumulation of body fat, loss of lean body tissue, and a decrease in aerobic capacity. Because much of the decline in bodily function seen in aging is analogous to that which accompanies a sedentary life style, one might hypothesize that this decline might be reversed with proper exercise. There are many physiological parameters that change with age. They include:

Musculoskeletal Changes

1. Muscle atrophy (reversible until approximately 60 years of age)
2. Decreased elasticity of connective tissue; dehydration of connective tissue and intervertebral disks
3. Bone demineralization resulting in postural deviations such as kyphosis and increased likelihood of fractures
4. Postural deviations which result from narrowing of the intervertebral disks, osteoporosis, and adaptive shortening of connective tissue

Cardio-Respiratory Changes

1. Decreased maximal heart rate
2. Decreased maximal oxygen uptake
3. Decreased vital capacity and expiratory volumes
4. Decreased minute ventilations

Additional Changes

1. Loss of balance due to degeneration of central nervous system

Many community colleges provide APE programs in retirement facilities. The primary role of the APE program in these facilities is to provide exercise programs that satisfy the physiological, social, and psychological needs of the senior adult. Although aging is not a disability, many physical limitations are associated with old age such as heart disease, arthritis, hypertension, and visual impairments. Thus, this population is more susceptible to injury during exercise and requires close supervision by assistants. Seniors are also more likely to be using medication than younger individuals.

Contraindicated Exercises

1. Isometric contractions of the arms, trunk, or legs.
2. Rapid twisting movements.
3. Ballistic stretching.
4. Standing toe touches.
5. Strenuous weight training.

Teaching Suggestions

1. Exercise programs for seniors should be progressive in design.
2. Do not overwork any joint or muscle group.
3. Do not stress activities that require static balance without vision or support.
4. Teach the whys of exercise.
5. Do not force people to participate.
6. Do not exacerbate existing conditions.
7. Treat participants as adults; validate their experience.
8. Present material slowly and in small steps.
9. Speak slowly and give good demonstrations.

Hearing Disorders

Hearing disorders may result in loss of amplitude (decibels) and pitch (hertz). The term "deaf" signifies that speech can not be heard even through amplification. Total deafness if rare. Hearing disorders are one of the most common chronic physical impairments in the United States.

The real handicap of a hearing disorder is the inability to communicate in the mainstream of society. New methods of standardized sign language, finger-spelling, and even lip reading have provided persons with hearing impairments greater opportunities for interacting with others. Therefore, more persons with hearing impairments are participating in regular physical education programs as opposed to adapted.

Types of Hearing Impairments

Congenital hearing impairment refers to the medical condition being present since birth. Adventitious hearing impairment refers to those conditions acquired later on in life.

Conductive deafness occurs when sound waves cannot be transmitted through either the outer or middle ear. The causes of this type of deafness could be the result of:

1. Congenital atresia
2. Middle ear infection due to
   a. Upper respiratory infection
   b. Diseased tonsils
   c. Adenoids
   d. Childhood diseases
   e. Otitis media
   f. Osteosclerosis

Sensorineural deafness occurs when sensory nerves of the inner ear are irreversibly damaged. A partial loss of equilibrium responses is frequently associated with sensorineural hearing losses.

Spectrum of Hearing Impairments				
Mild 20-30 db. loss	**Marginal** 30-40 db. loss Hearing Aid Language Deficiencies	**Moderate** 40-60 db. loss Special Education	**Severe** 60-75 db. loss "Educationally Deaf"	**Profound** 75+ db. loss Respond reflexively to loud sounds.

Characteristics of Persons with Hearing Impairments

1. **Balance (static or dynamic):** When there exists a sensorineural (inner ear) loss. However, may compensate through the use of visual and kinesthetic cues.
2. **Hyperactivity:** In order to maintain visual contact with all action occurring in the environment; boredom due to incomprehension.
3. **Socially Immature:** Due to delay in acquisition of speech and language; as children have difficulty grasping intricacies of team strategy.

Teaching Strategies

1. Do not have person face sun when instructing.
2. Do not talk while facing away from person. Circle formations are ideal.
3. Remove hearing aid during contact sports.
4. Keep hearing aid away from excessive moisture.
5. Use pictures and charts to reinforce demonstrations.
6. If balance dysfunction exists, supervise climbing and apparatus work
7. Do not exaggerate or raise voice when speaking to someone with a hearing aid. (Causes tension headaches.)
8. Assign teammate to act as a partner and inform participant of changes in the environment during group sports and activities.
9. Use visual cues (red flag, turn off lights) to get attention during activities.
10. Teach principles of equilibrium:
    a. Broad base of support.
    b. Lower center of gravity.
    c. Use of arms out to side.
    d. How to fall properly.
    e. Use of kneeling and sitting positions.
    f. Falling outside base of support.

Communicating with a Person Who is Hearing Impaired

1. **Get the person's attention before speaking.** A tap on the shoulder, a wave, or another visual signal usually does the trick.

2. **Key the person into the topic of discussion.** People with hearing impairments need to know what the subject of discussion is, in order to pick up words which help them follow the conversation. This is especially important for people who depend on oral communication.

3. **Speak slowly and clearly,** but do not yell, exaggerate, or over-pronounce. It's estimated that only 3 out of 10 spoken words are visible on the lips. Exaggeration and over-emphasis of words distort lip movements, making speech-reading more difficult. Try to enunciate each word, without force or tension. Short sentences are easier to understand than long ones.

4. **Look directly at the person** when speaking. Even a slight turn of your head can obscure their speech-reading view.

5. **Do not place anything in your mouth** when speaking. Mustaches that obscure the lips, smoking, pencil chewing, and putting your hands in front of your face make it difficult for persons with hearing impairments to follow what is being said.

6. **Maintain eye contact.** Eye contact conveys the feeling of direct communication. Even if an interpreter is present, continue to speak directly to the person with a hearing impairment. He/she will turn to the interpreter as needed.

7. **Avoid standing in front of a light source,** such as a window or bright light. The bright background and shadows created on the face make it almost impossible to speech-read.

8. **First repeat, then try to rephrase a thought** rather than again repeating the same words. If the person only missed one or two words the first time, one repetition usually will help. Particular combinations of lip movements sometimes are difficult for persons to speech-read. Don't be embarrassed to communicate by paper and pencil if necessary. Getting the message across is more important than the medium used.

9. **Use pantomime, body language, and facial expression** to help communicate. A lively speaker always is more interesting to watch.

10. **Be courteous** during conversation. If the telephone rings or someone knocks at the door, excuse yourself and tell the person that you are answering the phone or responding to the knock. Do not ignore the person and carry on a conversation with someone else while the person waits.

11. **Use open-ended question** which must be answered by more than "yes" or "no". Do not assume that the person has understood your message if he/she nods head in acknowledgment. Open-ended questions ensure that your information has been communicated.

Indicated Exercise Program

Although it is true that persons with hearing impairments frequently have special needs that could be met in an APE program, more often than not they do very well in mainstreamed physical education classes. For those with sensorineural hearing loss, developmental balance exercises are important due to the fact that the auditory organ has dual function of hearing and equilibrium. See Chapter 10 for a complete listing of balance progressions. Many persons with hearing impairments are also withdrawn socially from games, dances, and group activities; thus, an APE instructor may want to include activity choices that facilitate interaction and the development of appropriate social skills.

Learning Disabilities

The term learning disability (LD) has been used to describe a variety of problems in processing, retrieving, and storing visual and auditory information. Persons with a learning disability receive inaccurate information through their senses and/or have trouble processing that information. Educationally, LD results in a discrepancy between estimated IQ (average or above average) and academic performance (below average). It affects the ability to effectively use written or spoken language (dyslexia and aphasia, respectively).

The most commonly used definition is from The Education for All Handicapped Children Act of 1975 (Public Law 94-142):

The term "specific learning disabilities" refers to a disorder in one or more of the basic psychological processes involved in understanding or using language, spoken or written, which may manifest itself in imperfect ability to listen, speak, read, write, spell or do mathematical calculations. Such disorders include such conditions as perceptual handicaps, brain injury, minimal brain dysfunction, dyslexia and developmental aphasia. Such terms do not include learning problems which are primarily the result of visual, hearing or motor handicaps, of mental retardation, of emotional disturbances, or environmental, cultural or economic disadvantage.

Some people with LD (espeically children) have social skills problems because their perceptual problems make it difficult for them to understand others. A person who is unable to discriminate visually between the letters V and U might also be unable to see the differences between a friendly smile and a sarcastic smile. A person unable to discriminate between two different musical notes might be unable to hear the difference between a joking and a questioning voice. People with auditory handicaps work so hard to understand the words of a statement that they might ignore the nonverbal meaning. This confusion can cause people with LD to have difficulty fitting in with others. They might have trouble meeting people, working with others, talking to authority figures, and making friends.

Many people confuse mental retardation and learning disabilities. Mental retardation refers to subaverage cognition with concomitant deficits in adaptive behavior. Persons with LD have average or above-average IQ and function very well in regards to adaptive behavior. Many famous people have had a learning disability — Leonardo da Vinci, Hans Christian Anderson, and Albert Einstein. Can you name any current famous people who are learning disabled?

Theoretical Causes of Learning Disabilities

The following list of theories attempts to provide explanations of learning deficits. No theory completely explains learning disabilities; each theory offers only a partial explanation. One study found a genetic factor in about 20% of 500 case histories reviewed. The genetic link seems to be more common from male to male family members. There are a myriad of non-inherited dysfunction theories. Some of the present theories include brain injury, biochemical imbalances, maturational or developmental delay of the central nervous system, and sensorimotor dysfunctions.

1. **Minimal Brain Dysfunction** — Caused by damage to the brain at birth or during prenatal and post-natal periods. Lesions or scar tissue may be present.
2. **Neural Transmission Defects** — Caused by improper transmission of nerve impulses from one neuron to another across the synapse. Depending on the ratio of the chemicals, acetycholine and cholinesterase, which are present at the synapse, the nerve impulse may be transmitted either too slowly or too quickly.
3. **Maturational or Developmental Lag** — Relates mainly to the delay of the myelin sheath that encases the nerve fibers.
4. **Perceptual-Motor Match** — According to Kephard and Barsch, poor perceptual-motor-spatial abilities are related to learning deficits. Therefore, the ability to relate the self to time and space (balancing, laterality, directionality) should be remediated if learning deficits are to be overcome.

Other Etiological Factors

1. Prematurity.
2. Artificial food additives.
3. Malnutrition.
4. Infections (e.g., meningitis).
5. Toxins (e.g., lead).
6. Maternal drug abuse (e.g., cocaine)
7. Other suggested causes are: lack of oxygen at birth, premature birth, low birth weight, Caesarean birth, as well as food allergies.

Characteristics of Persons with Learning Disabilities

Learning disabilities can manifest itself in many forms. The following are but a few of the common areas of deficiencies.

Visual Perception

1. Figure-ground: Difficulty in seeing a specific image within a competing background.
2. Sequencing: Difficulty seeing figures in correct order; for example, seeing letters reversed.
3. Discrimination: Difficulty seeing the differences between two similar objects, such as the letters "c" and "e".
4. Spatial Awareness: Difficulty in judging distance, depth, and direction.
5. Ocular Tracking: Difficulty in tracking a moving object with the eyes.

Auditory Perception

1. Figure-ground: Difficulty in focusing on a specific image with competing background noise.
2. Memory: Difficulty remembering the a sequence of instructions.
3. Discrimination: Difficulty hearing the differences between two sounds or words; for example, "then" and "than."

Other Characteristics

1. hyperactivity
2. disorders of attention (Attention Deficit Disorder)
3. poor self-concept
4. impulsivity
5. apraxia (inability to execute coordinated, sequential movement skills)

Indicated Exercise Program

Activities found to be useful for the person with LD are: jogging, relaxation, perceptual-motor activities, highly structured, teacher-directed routines and noncompetitive games — all of which must be taught in a sequential fashion. In general, an exercise program for the person with LD should follow guidelines established for a total fitness program. Perceptual-motor training programs which are progressive in design have been developed by Jack Capon, Marianne Frostig, and Newell Kephart.

Although traditional perceptual-motor training has not been shown to conclusively remediate academic deficiencies, it can improve the perceptual-motor skills of the person with apraxia in physical education. Active learning games, developed by Dr. Bryant Cratty of UCLA, do help to reinforce the teaching of academic concepts.

Multiple Sclerosis

Definition

Multiple Sclerosis (MS) is a demyelinating disease of the brain and spinal cord. Myelin is the protective covering around nerve fibers which preserves the speed and intensity of the electrical nerve impulse. When MS is present, myelin is destroyed and replaced by scar tissue; consequently, nerve signals to and from the brain are distorted or blocked. The scarring plaques are usually present in the pyramidal and extrapyramidal tracts, cerebellum, brain stem, cerebral hemispheres, and optical pathways (Calliet, 1984). The lesions may occur in one or any combination of these sites. The damage to the upper motoneurons causes reflexes which are normally inhibited by these centers to become hyperactive. It strikes young adults, usually those between 20 and 40 years of age.

Clinical Picture

Symptoms include diplopia, nystagmus, ataxia, dysarthria, ipsilateral and bilateral paresis, and spasticity in the upper and lower extremities (Mankey, 1984). Demyelination also leads to early onset of fatigue. Optimal energy periods appear to be early mornings and evenings, and times of depressed metabolic rates. Heat, either external or internal, increases fatigue and worsens the symptoms. Shauf and Davis (1974) attributed the increased fatigue to a blockage of conducting fibers in the spinal cord. The prognosis for M.S. varies, but mortality statistics favor longevity.

Types of Multiple Sclerosis

Chronic Relapsing

This type is the most common form. It begins with symptoms of numbness, vertigo, and blindness. Episodes of symptoms lasting for several weeks tend to recur with increasing frequency. After 5 to 8 years, neurologic defects in the form of tremor, spasticity, speech or cerebellar incoordination persist. These abnormalities progress to the point that disabilities become irreversible.

Chronic Progressive

This type occurs most often in older persons and is characterized by gradual development and slow progression of spasticity and motor incapacity after 5 to 10 years. Death is usually caused by respiratory infection or some unrelated condition.

Acute M.S

This type is characterized by the rapid development and steady progression of paralytic symptoms, mainly affecting the function of the brain stem and often leading to death in several months. Curiously, patients who recover from an attack of acute MS are often free from subsequent attacks.

Indicated Exercise Program

1. Techniques of PNF should be employed as a primary means of restoration or maintenance of function. Hold-relax or contract-relax can be used to decrease spasticity and improve range of motion. Contractures are typically present in the plantarflexors, hamstrings, hip flexors, and hip adductors. If PNF relaxation techniques are not possible, then active or passive range of motion should be utilized. For strengthening, PNF slow-reversals should be employed to strengthen muscles (arms, trunk and legs) and facilitate reciprocal movement.

2. Swimming is recommended since active exercise may be performed more easily and with less fatigue than on land. The individual can sit in the shallow end and perform such movements as hip flexion, hip adduction, knee extension, knee flexion, dorsiflexion, ankle eversion, trunk flexion, and trunk extension. See Chapter 12 for specific exercises.

3. Developmental balance activities are usually the common program component for all participants with MS, although each person's ability will vary. See Chapter 10 for specific activities.

4. Due to balance deficits and muscular weakness (e.g., drop foot), gait training is usually instituted. This training may be initiated on the Kinetron and progress to the parallel bars. The participant with MS typically focuses on lifting one extremity through swing phase (dorsiflexion, knee flexion, and hip flexion). Characteristics of the MS (ataxic) gait include a wide base of support, drop foot, and circumducted hip during swing. Stationary leg cycling promotes reciprocal movements and strengthens the leg extensors.

5. Cardiovascular endurance is difficult to develop in participants with MS due to fatigue factors. Because excessive fatigue may induce some numbness or loss of function, participants should be cautious in over-exerting themselves. Interval training should be used so fatigue and over-heating are minimized.

6. Frenkel exercises were developed for conditions involving ataxia. They may be used with persons with MS and are described below:
   a. Lying position: Flexion and extension of each leg at the knee and hip joints. Abduction and adduction with the knee flexed; later, abduction and adduction with the knee extended.
   b. Flexion and extension of one knee at a time with the heel lifted off the mat.
   c. Knee flexed and heel paced upon some definite part of the other leg (e.g., patella). Change the heel from one position to another. Increase difficulty by calling for extension between different placings.

Spinal Cord Injury

Definition

Spinal cord injury involves damage to the soft neural tissue of the spinal cord. Once destroyed, nerve cells cannot be replaced. Spinal nerve fibers are unable to cross the site of injury and reestablish communication (unlike the peripheral nervous system). In contrast to some portions of the brain, the spinal cord has no alternate pathways or spare nerve cells that can take over the function of the damaged portion.

Damage to the spinal cord results in motor, sensory, and autonomic impairments. Sensory tracts (afferent) ascend through the cord and carry information from the sensory organs. If these tracts are injured, sensation (e.g., pain, temperature, touch) is lost below the level of injury. When motor tracts (efferent) are damaged, voluntary muscle control is lost below the level of injury. Autonomic deficits refer to damage to tracts which innervate smooth muscles of the body. Depending on the location and extent of damage, function of the viscera, heart, vasomotor responses, sweat glands, temperature control, bladder, and bowel may be impaired below the level of injury.

Etiology

Most traumatic injuries are associated with trauma to the boney structure of the vertebral column (e.g., contusion, crushing/compression, dislocation, fracture), while many non-traumatic injuries show little or no boney involvement. Non-traumatic injuries are generally associated with pathology such as infection, vascular disease, or degenerative disorders.

Types of Spinal Cord Injury

The degree of impairment as a result of spinal cord injury varies according to the level and extent of damage. Injuries are designated as complete or incomplete. Complete compression or transection of the spinal cord results in complete loss of any sensory, motor, and autonomic function below the level of injury. An incomplete injury results in a partial preservation of neurologic tracts, with any combination of motor, sensory, and autonomic function being retained. The prognosis will vary with incomplete injuries.

The level of the spinal cord injury is designated as the lowest nerve root segment with preserved function. For example, a person with a C-7 injury will have preserved function in the nerve root that exists below the seventh cervical vertebrae.

1. **Lower Motoneuron Lesion (LMN)** — Injury occurs below the first lumbar vertebrae (L-1). It is characterized by a loss of voluntary motor/sensory function and the presence of flaccid paralysis below the level of injury. Reflex arcs are destroyed, preventing involuntary spasms and hypertonic muscle.
2. **Upper Motoneuron Lesion (UMN)** — Injury occurs at or above the 12th thoracic vertebrae (T-12). It is characterized by the loss of voluntary control and the occurrence of spastic paralysis below the level of the injury. Spastic paralysis occurs when the reflex arc is intact below the level of injury; therefore, uninhibited stretch reflexes cause persistent involuntary muscular contractions and abnormally high tone.

Medical Complications (Upper Motoneuron Lesions)

1. Spasticity (hypertonic muscle, exaggerated stretch reflexes, clonus)
2. Contractures (hip flexors and adductors, hamstrings, plantarflexors)
3. Orthopedic deformities (e.g., scoliosis)
4. Inability to perspire below the level of lesion
5. Bladder infections
6. Bladder stones
7. Gastrointestinal disorders
8. Infections from catheterizations
9. Respiratory disorders
10. Autonomic dysreflexia (lesions above T-6)
11. Decubiti ulcers (pressure sores)

Spinal Nerves and Their Somatic Distribution

There are 31 pairs (right and left) of spinal nerves. Each spinal nerve exits between two adjacent vertebrae through the intervertebral foramen. There are eight cervical (C), 12 thoracic (T), five lumbar (L), five sacral (S), and one coccygeal (Cx) pair of spinal nerves. Each spinal nerve is identified according to its exit zone (C, T, L, S, or Cx) and its number in the area. For example, spinal nerve T-9 exits through the intervertebral foramen formed by thoracic vertebrae 9 and 10 (Smith, 1974). There are eight nerves that exit the cervical spine, but only seven cervical vertebrae. The first through the seventh nerves exit above the cervical vertebra and above the first thoracic vertebra. The first thoracic nerve then exits below the first thoracic vertebra. (Hoppenfeld, 1976. The chart on the right details this distribution.

Spinal Nerves	Plexus	Somatic Distribution
C-1	———	Some muscles of the head and throat.
2	Cervical Plexus	Some muscles of the throat, neck, and shoulder joint.
3		
4		
5		
6		
7	Brachial Plexus	Muscles of the shoulder girdle and shoulder joint.
8		
T-1		Muscles of the upper extremity.
T-2 - T-11	No Plexus	Muscles of the trunk.
T-12		Muscles of the hip joint.
L-1	Lumbar Plexus	Anterior and medial muscles of the hip and knee joints.
2		
3		
4		
5		
S-1	Sacral Plexus	Muscles of the knee and ankle joints and the foot.
2		
3		

Adapted from Smith, 1974

Predicted Functional Potential According to Level of Lesion

C-5	Partial strength of all shoulder motions Electric chair Attendant for help with ADL Elbow flexion
C-6	Normal shoulder, elbow flexion Wrist extension Minimal assistance with transfer
C-7	Independent transfers Manual wheelchair Elbow extension Finger extension
T-1	Normal arms and hands Totally independent in most activities
T-6	Upper trunk muscles Inadequate bronchial hygiene Weak cough Limited chest expansion
T-6 to T-12	Potential for community ambulation with braces
T-12	Thorax, abdomen, and low back muscles
L-2 to L-5	Ambulation with the use of braces
L-4	Hip flexion Knee extension
L-5	Partial strength of hip motions with normal flexion Partial strength of ankle and foot motion

Indicated Exercise Program

1. Provide passive range of motion for paralyzed muscle groups (e.g., plantar-flexors, hamstrings, hip flexors and adductors) and active range of motion for innervated muscle groups.
2. Strengthen and hypertrophy those muscles that are suitable substitutes for others that are permanently weakened or paralyzed (e.g., shoulder internal rotators for forearm pronators). A combination of techniques can be utilized, including PNF, manual resistance, and PRE.

3. Provide training for cardiovascular endurance (see protocol and precautions for arm crank ergometry in Chapter 8 — Assessment and Programming for Cardiovascular Endurance).
4. Wheelchair dips (if elbow extension present) prevent decubiti ulcers by allowing circulation. Lift buttocks off chair by extending at elbow and hold 60 seconds.
5. If possible, use standing frame or parallel bars to help prevent contractures, disuse osteoporosis, and maintain any residual strength in legs. It may be possible to use one of the crutch gait patterns (Chapter 9 — Assessment and Programming for Gait).
6. Encourage sitting balance activities (Chapter 10).
7. Development of the triceps (elbow extension) is extremely important in facilitating transfers, gait training, and wheelchair propulsion. In addition, strengthening of the latissimus dorsi is highly indicated (shoulder adduction) for persons with spinal cord injury. This muscle bridges the paralyzed parts of the body with the nonparalyzed muscles and assists in sitting balance and postural awareness.

Catheters

In many instances of spinal cord injury, the bladder becomes neurogenic (paralyzed). This condition may necessitate the use of a catheter, a device used for draining the urine from the bladder. The types of catheters worn by individuals include:

1. Indwelling Urethral
2. Suprapubic
3. External (condom)

Occasionally, exercise positions will have to be modified so as not to interfere with the functioning of these devices. It is suggested that the instructor obtain this information during the initial evaluation with the participant.

Autonomic Dysreflexia

Autonomic dysreflexia occurs in individuals with spinal cord lesions above T-6. It is considered an acute emergency requiring immediate medical attention. Early recognition of dysreflexic symptoms is essential in order to prevent bleeding in or near the brain (cerebrovascular accident). The symptoms include the following (Larson & Snobl, 1978):

1. Pounding headache (due to severe rise in blood pressure)
2. Profuse sweating above the level of injury
3. Goose bumps
4. Splotching of the skin
5. Nasal obstruction

The causes for dysreflexia vary, the most common being over-distention of the bladder (blocked catheter), severe spasms, infection, kidney stones, distention of the bowel, or pressure sores.

If the person is in a horizontal position when the dysreflexia occurs, elevate the head or bring the body to a sitting position as quickly as possible to induce a drop in blood pressure. The catheter for the bladder should be immediately checked for blockages (e.g., kinks in the tubing, overfull bag, clamps which have not been removed, blocked inlets to the leg bag). Do not forget to call the paramedics immediately.

Wheelchair Athletic Injuries — Causes & Prevention

Soft Tissue Injuries

Causes

1. Tearing and overstretching of ligaments (falls, physical contact)
2. Chronic overuse of muscles and tendons
3. Overexertion without proper warm-up

Prevention

1. Routine stretching, warm-up and cool-down for each workout
2. Slowly progress strengthening/conditioning program — don't jump into it at once
3. Preventive taping, splinting for better stabilization/protection of old injuries

Blisters

Causes

1. Traction or irritation of skin in contact with wheelchair rim
2. Irritation of skin at top of seat post or back of wheelchair upholstery

Prevention

1. Encourage callous formation as initial protection
2. Taping of fingers
3. Wearing gloves
4. Padding over seat post area
5. Wear shirt between skin and wheelchair back

Abrasions/Lacerations/Cuts

Causes

1. Fingers, thumbs in contact with brakes or metal edge of arm rest socket or push rim
2. Inner arm in contact with larger tires of track chair on downstroke
3. Chair contact (basketball) trapping fingers between wheels

Prevention

1. Remove brakes
2. Use arm rests or file off sockets for arm rests
3. Wear clothing or protective covering for upper arms
4. Camber wheels for wheelchair basketball chairs

Decubitus/Pressure Areas (mainly a problem for those without sensation)

Causes

1. Shear forces and pressure over sacrum and buttocks with friction on chair
2. Track wheelchair design with knees higher than buttocks may contribute
3. Sweat, moisture in combination with shear forces

Prevention

1. Adequate cushioning and padding for buttocks
2. Frequent skin checks over buttocks and sacrum
3. Shifting weight to relieve pressure intermittently
4. Good nutrition and hygiene
5. Clothing that absorbs moisture

Temperature Regulation Disorders

Causes

1. Exposure to hot sun/heat or cold in absence of temperature control or sweating mechanisms
2. Inadequate fluid intake/excessive water loss

Prevention

1. Wear adequate clothing for protection in hot and cold weather (insulation)
2. Replace fluids — drink water
3. Assist with heat convection — cool towels over body surfaces or spray bottle
4. Minimize exposure — seek shade and cover

Visual Impairments

All definitions of visual impairments refer to how well the individual can see even with the best of corrective lenses. Normal vision is technically referred to as 20/20. This numerical ratio is interpreted as the ability to see at 20 feet what the normal eye can see at 20 feet. A person is considered partially sighted or visually impaired if visual acuity is 20/70 or less with correction - interpreted as the ability to see at 20 feet what the normal eye can see at 70 feet. Visual acuity is measured with a Snellen Chart (lines of letters which become smaller with each line). Over 75% of persons with visual impairments in the United States have some usable vision.

Visual impairments take many forms. Some may see a tiny spot of the visual field and even though the spot of vision is 20/20, they may be considered legally blind. Fuzzy vision, peripheral vision, tunnel vision make the description of visual impairment difficult to understand. The amount of light and contrasts in the environment influences visual ability in persons with impairments. For example, a person may not need a guide during daylight hours because contrasts are sufficient to permit independent movement. However, during the evening or in a dark room such as a theater, a sighted guide may be necessary because no contrasts are available.

Visual impairments are usually classified in the following manner (Sherrill, 1986):

1. **20/200 — legally blind**: The ability to see at 20 feet what persons with normal vision can see at 200 feet.
2. **5/200 to 10/200 — travel vision**: The ability to see at 5 to 10 feet what persons with normal vision see at 200 feet.
3. **3/200 to 5/200 — motion perception**: The ability to see at 3 to 5 feet what persons with normal vision can see at 200 feet. Refers primarily to the ability to detect motion.
4. **Less than 3/200 — light perception**: The ability to detect a bright light from 3 feet, but inability to detect movement of a hand at the same distance.
5. **Lack of visual perception — total blindness**: Inability to detect a bright light that is shown directly into the eye.

Common Types and Etiology

1. **Macula Degeneration** — The macula is located in the central portion of the retina. Degeneration affects central vision, but the person maintains good peripheral vision. Usually this condition does not progress to total blindness.
2. **Glaucoma** — Excessive high pressure within the eyeball, creating tunnel vision.
3. **Cataracts** — A clouding of the cornea. The incidence of blindness from cataracts has decreased due to surgical techniques.
4. **Retinitis Pigmentos**a — An inherited condition in which the rod-shaped cells in the retina degenerate. This disorder leads to total blindness.
5. **Diabetic Retinopathy** — Because diabetes can induce vascular changes, the retina is particularly susceptible to hemorrhage, scarring, and loss of vision.
6. **Stroke** — Blindness can be caused by lack of blood supply to the visual cortex located in the occipital lobe. Blindness occasionally occurs in stroke cases where the person is only capable of seeing out of one side of each eye (hemianopsia).
7. **Refractory Errors** — This includes farsightedness, nearsightedness, and astigmatism.
8. Blindness can be a result of venereal disease, the aging process, trauma causing detached retina, tumors, or exposure to bright light (e.g., sun, welding light).

Characteristics

The functional ability of a person who is blind or visually impaired varies, depending upon age of onset and whether the impairment is total or partial. A person who is visually impaired or has some perception of form and light may be completely independent with full use of his/her other senses. With proper training in the use of braille, large type books, tape recorders, new technological equipment and good mobility skills, individuals who are blind can be as functionally independent as their community will allow. Individuals who have been totally blind since birth do not have any visual memory and therefore learn to use their intact senses to perceive what others see. Some individuals with visual impairments may display mannerisms such as eye-poking or rocking, usually due to a need for physical stimulation.

Techniques for Guiding a Person with Visual Impairment

1. Making contact — Lightly brush forearms with the person so he/she can find the back of your arm, proximal to the elbow. Keep your elbow flexed to 90 degrees. This position enables the person to be at your side but about a half-step behind.
2. Familiarize the person to the environment. When you give directions, give them according to the way the person is facing — left or right. When entering a room, indicate number of people present, size of room, and general description.
3. Pause before any stairs or curbs. Describe the height of the step up or down.
4. When approaching a door, inform the person whether the door will swing "away" or "toward" him/her and if it opens to the left or right. Swing the door open as far as possible and whisk the person through before it swings shut.
5. When seating, deposit the person at the back of the chair and allow him/her to seat himself/herself. Alternate method: back person up into the seat until the calves touch.
6. If going through a narrow passageway, keep your elbow flexed, but internally rotate your shoulder, placing your arm behind your back. The person will then slide the hand from the back of your bicep to the middle of the forearm and step directly behind you.

Indicated Exercise Program

It is recommended that each person with visual impairments have a medical verification completed by an ophthalmologist. These doctors have differing philosophies regarding physical activities for persons with visually impaired (e.g., bending over during exercise, putting the face in the water when swimming). Therefore, a phone call to the attending eye care specialist would be useful, **especially** in the case of diabetic retinopathy.

The mode of exercise may vary depending on the degree of vision remaining and risk of injury to the eye. If an individual has no functional vision, his/her choice of physical activities may actually expand without fear of further deterioration. For a discussion of exercise precautions and contraindications regarding the eye, see section on diabetic retinopathy under Diabetes of this chapter.

1. **Encourage cardiovascular endurance.** The person with visual impairments rarely gets an opportunity to engage in aerobic activities due to the amount of supervision or guiding required and thus evidence low endurance. Utilize stationary cycling, low-intensity rowing on a row machine, tandem cycling, folk and square dance, aerobic dance, swimming, and jogging. If an indoor track is available, a guide wire can assist with independent locomotion. On an outdoor track, a sighted guide can assist with walking or jogging by simply touching forearms occasionally as the two move side-by-side; another method is to extend a short rope between the two persons to maintain contact and control. Swimming is an ideal activity because it builds strength and cardiovascular endurance while requiring minimal assistance from a partner. Swimming is easily adaptable as buoys and rope lanes prevent a individual from straying out of a lane while swimming laps. A "bonker" (soft sponge ball attached to a long wooden dowel) may be used to tap the swimmer on the head and signal the edge of the pool and end of the lap.

2. **Development individual sport activities and leisure skills that have life-long, carry-over value.** Because of equipment adaptations in sports such as archery, persons with visual impairments are able to recreate and compete alongside sighted persons. Teaching adaptations have also broadened sports participation by persons with visual impairments; for example, snow skiing may be accomplished through the use of a sighted guide and auditory input. Folk dancing may be performed by mingling sighted partners with non-sighted partners. Circle formations are especially helpful in providing spatial orientation during dance steps.

3. **Postural exercises may need to be prescribed for lordosis, ptosis, kyphosis.**

4. **Goal ball**, a modified form of soccer played while positioned on the hands and knees, is a very popular sport created for athletes with visual impairments. It is played on an indoor gymnasium with two teams and an audible ball. National competitions are held each year. See Chapter 14 for a more detailed description of the game.

A person desiring to participate in competitive sports for athletes with visual impairments should write to the United States Association for Blind Athletes, 33 N. Institute Street, Brown Hall, Suite 015, Colorado Springs, CO 80903, for membership information and the yearly calendar for track and field, goal ball, snow skiing, and archery competitions.

Study Questions / Learning Activities

1. Select 2 disabilities found within this chapter and read each accompanying section. Next observe your instructor assess two persons, each with one of these disabilities. Consult with your instructor after the assessments are completed and assist him/her in developing an individualized exercise program for the two individuals. Note how each individual varies in ability and how their individualized exercise programs differ from the general descriptions provided in this chapter.

2. Write a case study on a participant in your APE program. Interview the selected participant to obtain his/her: (1) medical history since the onset of the disability; (2) lifestyle changes, if any; (3) past and current recreational/ sport pursuits; any medications affecting exercise performance; (4) long and short term physical activity goals; (5) assessment information; and (6) indicated exercise program.

3. Contact local agencies (e.g., Multiple Sclerosis Society, United Cerebral Palsy, Arthritis Foundation, Juvenile Diabetes Foundation) and have a representative visit your APE program and present a lecture on the disability they serve as an advocate for. These agencies may also loan informative videos to your program for supplementing the training of assistants. In addition, request free literature from the agencies in order to set up a mini-library for the APE program or for your own personal files.

4. Contact the same local agencies as above and inquire about what types of recreation and sport activities they sponsor for persons with disabilities. Attend one of their sponsored events.

5. Read through this chapter and write down unfamiliar terms on separate note-cards. Look up the definitions of these terms and write them on the back of the notecards. Use these flash cards in quiz-types games with the group of assistants.

References

American Heart Association (1986, 3rd ed.). *Guidelines for exercise testing and prescription.* Philadelphia: Lea and Febiger.

American Heart Association. Subcommittee on Exercise/Cardiac Rehabilitation (1981). Statement on exercise. *Circulation*, 64, 1302A.

Basmajian, J. V. (1977). *Therapeutic exercise.* Baltimore: Waverly Press.

Bleck, E. E. (1975). *Physically handicapped children — A medical atlas for teachers.* San Francisco: Grune and Stratton.

Bullock, E. A. (1974). Later stages of rehabilitation in hemiplegics. *Physiotherapy, 60,* 370-374.

Cooper, I. S. (1979). *Living with chronic neurologic disease*. New York: Norton and Co.

Daniels, A., & Davies, E. (1977). *Adapted physical education* (3rd edition). New York: Harper and Row.

Epilepsy Foundation of America (1981). *Epilepsy handbook for teachers and nurses*. 1612 30th Street, San Diego, CA, 92101.

Frenkel, L., & Richard, B. B. (1977). *Be alive as long as you live.* Charleston: Preventicare Publications.

French, R., & Jansma, P. (1982). *Special physical education.* Columbus: Merrill Publishing.

Glaser, R. M., Sawka, M. N., Durbin, R. J., Foley, D. M., & Suryaprasad, A. G. (1981). Exercise program for wheelchair activity. *American Journal of Physical Medicine, 60*(2), 67-75.

Graham, C., & Lasko-McCarthey, P. (1990). Exercise options for persons with diabetic complications. *Diabetes Educator, 16*(3), 212-220.

Greenlee, G. (1987). Exercise options for patients with reinopathy and peripheral vascular disease. *Practical Diabetology, 6*(4), 9-11.

Haring, N. (1982). *Exceptional children and youth* (3rd edition). Columbus: Merrill Publishing.

Hollander, J. (1976). *The arthritis handbook.* West Point: Merck, Hape, and Dohme Publishing.

Jennett, B. (1975). Outcome after severe brain damage. A practical scale. *Lancet, 1,* 480-483.

Knopf, K. G., & Downs, S. (1988). *Fitness over fifty.* Dubuque: Kendall-Hunt.

Lavigne, J. *Home exercises for patients with Parkinson's Disease.* The American Parkinson Disease Association.

Mason, E., & Dando, H. (1975). *Corrected therapy and adapted physical education.* Chillicothe, Ohio: American Corrective Therapy Association.

Pollock, M. L., Miller, H. S., Linnerud, A. C., Laughridge, E., Coleman, E., & Alexander, E. (1974). Arm pedaling as an endurance training regimen for the disabled. *Archives of Physical Medicine and Rehabilitation, 55,* 252-261.

Sager, K. (1984). Exercises to activate seniors. *Physician and Sportsmedicine, 12*(5), 144-151.

Schauf, C. L., & Davis, F. A. (1974). Impulse conduction in multiple sclerosis: A theoretical basis for modification by temperature and pharmacological agents. *Journal of Neurology, Neurosurgery, and Psychology, 37,* 152-161.

Umphred, D. A. (1985). *Neurological rehabilitation.* St. Loius: C. V. Mosby.

14

Sports Participation

James Burke, Director,
Fitness Clinic for the Physically Disabled
San Diego State University

Stroke Technique for Wheelchair Sports

Before engaging in wheelchair actvities, the instructor must teach the essentials of a stroke, using a three-step progression:

1. Grasp the push rims or the push rims and tires on the wheel at the point below the shoulders.
2. Push the wheels forward with both hands moving simultaneously, evenly and fluidly.
3. Maintain contact with the push rims after the forward stroke is finished by sliding hands up the push rims to the starting position. By maintaining contact with the push rims, one increases the efficiency of the stroke.

Teaching Progression for Wheelchair Mobility

Pushing a Straight Line

1. On a flat surface, stroke wheels with both hands at the same time in a long fluid motion. If hands do not stroke at the same time, the chair will move erratically.
2. On sloped surfaces, push harder on the wheel which is lowest on the slope. This will counteract the effects of the slope.

Turning the Chair

1. Turing right or left may be accomplished by applying pressure on the push rim which faces the direction you wish to move in, and stroking the opposite wheel more aggressively.
2. In a faster situation, one may need to slow the chair before turning by applying pressure equally to both push rims. As the turn approaches, simply press harder on the wheel which faces the direction you wish to move in, and stroke the opposite wheel.

Cutting (Sharp Turns) in a Wheelchair

A technique used often in wheelchair basketball and tennis. Grab the push rims (or the push rim and tire) which face the direction you wish to cut in first, then very aggressively push the opposite wheel. This progression must be done extremely quickly to be effective.

Ascending and Descending Ramps

1. When ascending a ramp of any height, one must move his/her center of gravity forward to maintain constant contact of all four wheels on the surface. The stroke here becomes shorter and quicker.
2. When descending a ramp, one must lean back against the backrest of the chair. This position will keep the bulk of the individual's body weight to the rear of the chair and help in maintaining contact with all four wheels of the chair to the surface.

The Wheelie

Fear of falling backwards out of the chair often affects the proper learning of this skill.

1. First it is important for the person to feel the degree ot tilt in either direction beyond where balance is established. A spotter whom the person trusts actively finds these points.
2. Wheelie progression.
    a) With the person in a wheelie beyond the balance point, the spotter should ask the person to lean the torso forward.
    b) With the person in a wheelie below the balance point, the spotter should ask the person to lean back.
    c) The person should try now to control the wheelie, with the spotter preventing a fall, by using the wheels. By very quickly pushing the wheels forward and leaning back, one may be able to bring front casters off the ground. By leaning forward and pulling the wheels back toward the body, one may bring the front casters toward the ground.
    d) A combination of these movements will enable the person to hold his/her wheelie.

Characteristics of a Sports Wheelchair

Wheels
- May be cambered to increase stability of the chair without sacrificing its turning ability.
- The axle may be moved forward or backward to adjust the turning angle of the chair or to increase its stability. The closer the axles are to the front of the chair, the easier it is to turn. This position does reduce stability.
- The axle plate or axle position may be raised or lowered, assisting the posture of the person. A person with poor sitting balance will benefit by lowering the wheelchair seat. This position is accomplished by raising the axle or axle plates.
- The hubs of most sport chairs are equipped with quick release axles, allowing the wheels to be removed easily.

Backrest
- Most sport chairs have backrests with push handles available on request. This is entirely up to the individual.
- Most backrests are adjustable. They can be lowered or raised depending on the posture of the person.

Frame
- Folding frame chairs are very useful to a person who must transfer to and from a car. However, the ride in a folding chair is usually not as smooth as a rigid frame chair.
- Rigid frame chairs do sacrifice convenience and practicality. The ride in a rigid chair is much smoother. There is less play in a rigid frame. Folding chairs are rarely used in athletics because of the superiority of the rigid chair's ride.

Casters
- There are forked casters and pin casters. Forked casters are smoother and negotiate obstacles better. Pin casters turn much faster and are more desirable on a playing court.

For a more detailed description of how to order a racing chair and select components, see the article by Cooper (1988) at the end of this chapter.

Wheelchair   Basketball

Rules (Source: National Wheelchair Basketball Association)

Wheelchair basketball is played in accordance with NCAA rules with very few exceptions. These exceptions are:

1. **Player eligibility** is limited to those individuals who, because of permanent severe leg disability or paralysis of the lower portion of the body, would be prevented from playing stand-up basketball.
2. **Wheelchair.** The height of the seat must not exceed 21 inches from the floor. Foot platforms must be 4 and 7/8ths inches from the floor with seat

cushions permitted only for therapeutic reasons. Each chair must be equipped with a heel strap of 1 and 1/2 inch width. The chair is considered a part of the player. General rules of contact in regular and stand-up basketball (charging, blocking, etc.) apply to wheelchair basketball.

3. **Jump Ball**. For any jump ball, each jumper shall remain firmly seated in his chair. He cannot lift his buttocks off the seat by use of arm, leg or force of movement. The jumper must be in the jumping circle at a 45 degree angle to his own basket.

4. **Dribbling**. A player may wheel the chair and bounce the ball simultaneously just as a man may run and bounce the ball simultaneously in regular basketball. In addition, a man with the ball in his possession can take no more than two consecutive pushes, with one or both hands, in either direction. If he has taken two pushes, he must shoot, pass or bounce the ball before pushing again. The latter can be repeated again as there isn't any double dribble violation. Three or more consecutive pushes with the ball in his possession constitutes a traveling violation.

5. **Loss of Ball**. If a man in possession of the ball makes any physical contact with the floor or tilts his chair so far forward that the footrests touch or as far backwards that the safety casters touch the floor, it is a violation and the ball is awarded to the other team.

6. **Falling Out of a Chair**. If a competitor falls out of his chair, or if his chair becomes inoperable during play, the officials will immediately suspend play if there is any chance of danger to the fallen player. If not, the officials will withhold their whistles until the particular play in progress has been completed. If a player falls out of his chair to gain possession of the ball, the ball is awarded to the opposing team.

7. **Time Limits**. An offensive player cannot remain more than 5 seconds in the free throw lane while his team is in possession of the ball in his front court.

8. **Out of Bounds**. A player is considered out of bounds when he or any part of his wheelchair touches the floor on or outside the boundary.

9. **Physical Advantage Foul**. Because of the varying causes and degrees of disability among participants, a basic rule of keeping firmly seated in the wheelchair at all times and not using a functional leg or leg stump for physical advantage over an opponent, is strictly enforced. An infraction of this rule (rebound, jump ball, etc.) constitutes a physical advantage foul. It is so recorded in the official score book. Three such fouls disqualify a player from the game. A free throw is awarded and the ball is given to the opposing team, out of bounds.

10. **Back Court Foul**. A defensive player who commits a personal foul in his opponent's back court shall be charged with a back court foul. The offended player shall be awarded two (2) free throws.

Equipment

1. Axles of the wheelchairs should be moved forward.
2. Footrests should consist of rowbars with rollers in order to prevent a player from being dumped.
3. Wheelchair seats are deep and angled (knees are higher than hips) to facilitate balance.

Basic Game Strategy

1. **Offense**. On offense work for the *inside shot*. The *outside shot* (12-15 ft. range) has a much lower success percentage. To get in position for the inside shot, set picks and screens.
2. **Defense**. Man-to-man defense is generally preferable for defense because it is easier to screen out for position. Younger, more inexperienced teams may use a zone defense.

Skills to be Mastered

1. **Wheelchair Mobility**. (See section on Teaching Progression for Wheelchair Mobility.)
2. **Dribbling**.
   a. Basic hand placement: fingers are spread and the elbow is stationary. Action is in the wrist and fingers.
   b. Practice stationary dribbling 6-8 times without looking, using both right and left hands.
   c. Dribble a half circle in front of the chair, let to right and right to left. Practice this maneuver with both right and left hands. Balance may pose a problem for some individuals.
   d. Basic dribble: involves one bounce, then placement of ball in lap and 2 pushes.
   e. Continuous dribble while pushing: dribble up and down the court with one hand. Use a high bounce with one hand push for long distances. Cross-lateral dribble involves continuous dribbling using both the right and left hands.
3. **Ball pick up using the rim of the wheelchair**.
   Partner rolls the ball down the court. The ball is approached and scooped up against the wheel rim, bringing it up to the top where it can be placed in the lap and dribbled. Practice should take place with both the right and left hands.
4. **Passing/receiving from a stationary wheelchair**. (Note reaction of wheelchair).
   a. Two-handed chest pass.
   b. Baseball pass, right and left (sidearm).
   c. Shovel pass (underhand).
   d. Bounce pass.
   e. Overhead lob.
   f. Hook pass.
5. **Passing/receiving from a moving wheelchair**.
   a. Forward moving.
   b. Backward moving (more advanced skill).
6. **Precaution**.
   No passing from a turning wheelchair. This is regarded as a low percentage pass and is considered a safety risk.
7. **Wheelchair positioning to receive pass**.

8. **Shooting and release of ball.**
    a. Wheelchair positioning for angles.
    b. Free throw.
    c. Lay ups, right and left side.
    d. Two-handed set shot.
    e. One-handed set shot (stationary and moving to position).
    f. Moving lay up, left and right side, using 2-man (in lines) with rebound recovery.
    g. Fast break (3-man).

Drills

1. Wheelchair mobility. (See section on Teaching Progression for Wheelchair Mobility)
2. Half court sprints.
3. Speed pushing (in lines with athletes at 10 ft. intervals): free throw to baseline, half court to baseline, free throw at opposite end to baseline, baseline to baseline. Include pivots in this drill, alternating turning right and left.
4. Push backwards across court lengths to refine symmetry of push, not for speed.
5. Relay races.
6. Shuttle runs.
7. Sprint races.
8. Slalom courses with stops and turns (right and left), spins, backward pushing, and sprints. May include dual and team races, as well as "follow-the-leader".
9. Cutting in and out of traffic cones.
10. Pass at a wall target while sitting stationary.
11. Pass at a wall target with a moving wheelchair (forward and lateral movement; no backward movement due to safety hazard).
12. Stationary passing and receiving (all types).
13. Incorporate mobile receiver with stationary passer and vice versa.
14. Moving passers and receivers with two moving lines with partners passing and receiving.
15. Caterpillar.
16. Shoot around: athletes shooting in pairs.
17. Shooting from a moving wheelchair.
18. Timing, wheelchair push/dribble/lay up.
19. Wheelchair moving shot (2 hands, 1 hand).

Wheelchair   Tennis

Rules

1. Two bounces are used in wheelchair tennis. A ball may hit the ground twice before being returned. The second bounce can land anywhere. Only the first bounce must land in the playing court. Also, the athlete may choose to hit the ball on either bounce.

2. The services must be accomplished with the rear wheels behind the baseline. Chair faults will be implemented if the rear wheels touch or cross the baseline. before the racket makes contact with the ball.
3. Open and "C" division servers may not bounce the ball on the ground for service. In the "Novice" division a bounce serve may be used.
4. The wheelchair shall be forbidden to touch the net or the ground within an opponent's court at anytime while the ball is in play.
5. If the ball touches the player or his chair, the player loses the point. This holds true only if the player is in the playing court. In essence, the chair is considered to be part of the person.
6. If the person is out-of-bounds and is struck by the ball, the ball is called out only if the player makes no attempt to hit the ball or tries to get away from the ball. If the ball hits the player's racket, then the ball is good. If the player is inside the playing court or is touching the line and the ball hits him, then the ball is good even if the player feels the ball would go out.
7. A player cannot intentionally jump out of his chair to hit or retrieve a ball, nor can he stand up in his chair to serve a ball. This rule is a judgment call and is to be determined by a court umpire. If a player unintentionally leaves the chair to make a play, no penalty is assessed.
8. In order to protect playing surfaces, the tournament officials may not allow a person to participate with black tires or anything which will mark the court.
9. A "maintenance delay" is a delay in the progress of a match due to a malfunction of a wheelchair, prosthesis or assistive device. Such delay must be requested by the player, granted by the umpire at the match, and shall not exceed 5 minutes. Only two such delays may be granted for each player for each match.

Skills to be Mastered

1. **Wheelchair Mobility.**
   Since lack of maneuverability is one of the common problems in wheelchair tennis, it is important that athletes develop skill in moving to and from various court positions.
2. **Forward Mobility.**
   To move forwards to a ball, both wheels of the chair are pushed evenly. The wheel on the side of the racket hand can be pushed either by using the base of the thumb or by pushing with the lower forearm.
3. **Backwards Mobility.**
   To move backwards from a ball, both wheels of the chair are pulled evenly.
4. **Lateral Mobility.**
   a. To move to the left, push the right wheel and either hold or pull the left wheel.
   b. To move to the right, push the left wheel and either hold or pull the right wheel.
   c. Turning can be achieved faster when traveling backwards since the small steering wheels are then at the opposite or back end of the chair to the direction of travel.

    d.   After playing a backhand shot (for a right-handed person), the right-hand side of the chair faces the net. To straighten up quickly, pull the right wheel with the left hand, and then push the left wheel with the left hand. The first movement can be done while executing the stroke or follow-through.

5. **Stopping.**
Sudden stopping of forward momentum is necessary to be able to quickly return to the best position on court, and it is achieved by leaning slightly backwards in the chair while gripping both wheels.

6. **Forehand Grip and Swing.**

7. **Backhand Grip and Swing.**

8. **Overhand and Underhand Serve.**

9. **Volley.**

Drills

1. **Familiarization with equipment (racket, ball, and wheelchair).**

2. **Wheelchair mobility and court positions.**

3. **Forehand Swing.**
    a.   Practice swing without ball.
    b.   Assistants toss the tennis ball from the service line to the athletes positioned on the baseline (same side of court). Athletes should be positioned on the right, middle and left sides of the baseline.
    c.   Assistants toss the tennis ball across the net to the athletes positioned on the baseline (opposite side of court).
    d.   Assistants hit the tennis ball across the net to the athletes positioned on the baseline (opposite side of court).
    e.   Assistants rally cross-court with athletes across the net from baseline.
    f.   Assistants rally down the line with athletes across the net from baseline.
    g.   Assistants alternate cross-court and down-the-line with athletes from across the net.
    h.   Athletes rally with one another from across the net.

4. **Backhand Swing.**
Follow same drills for #3.

5. **Overhand and Underhand Serve.**
    a.   Use a side on "stance" for the serve as this gives the ball better direction and the action of the arm is stronger in this position.
    b.   Practice the ball toss without the racket.
    c.   Serves should first be practiced without the ball.
    d.   The conventional overhand serve may need to be adapted due to the design of the wheelchair (full backswing may not be possible). Start by putting the racket down the back and then bring it forward over the head with the arm fully extended, making contact with the ball directly over the chair. The serve ends with a shortened follow through. The underhand serve can be used with beginners or those with limited arm strength. Practice serving on the service line first, then move to the baseline.
    e.   Practice serving into either of the opposite service areas.

Goalball for Persons with Visual Impairments

Framework for Goalball

A game is played by three players on each of two teams. The game is conducted on the floor of a gymnasium within a rectangular court which is divided into two halves by a center line (see court diagram in Appendix H). The goals are erected at both ends. The game is to be played with a bell ball. The object of the game is for each team to roll the ball across the opponent's goal line, while the other team attempts to prevent this from happening.

Skills to be Mastered — Offense

1. **Throwing.** (stems from bowling style roll/throw)
   a. Legs: 1 to 5 step approach (depending on where they are on the court.
   b. Two-handed hold on the ball, backswing.
   c. From backswing, beginning forward movement of shoulder joint, plenty of follow-through after ball release.
   d. Must coordinate with foot movement.
2. **Passing.**
   a. Moving the ball between three players after one player has thrown ball two times consecutively.
   b. Note: Communication between players on offense consists of verbal, finger-snapping, tapping on the floor, etc.
3. **Localizing.**
   a. Ability to distinguish ball noise from distracting sounds.
   b. Able to distinguish other players' positions on the court.

Skills to be Mastered — Defense

1. **Lunge:** Diving movement from a two-footed erect standing or squatting position to a prone position. Incorporates full body extension.
2. **Auditory.**
   a. Ability to track the sound of the ball.
   b. Ability to utilize cues from teammates.
   c. Auditory discrimination.
   d. Ability to lunge in the right direction at the right time.
   e. Ability to coordinate specific defensive patterns with teammates; i.e., lunging in same direction, etc.

Skills to be Mastered — Orientation

All lines on court are marked off by rope covered with tape so the goalball players can orient themselves in their area of the court. Players must know where they are on the court by feeling the lines or the goal case around them.

Skills to be Mastered — Mobility

When players are on the court, they play in specific areas. Two back players are located at the 1.50m lines, and one center player is stationed at the .50m line.

Safety Considerations

1. Bicycle helmet for head.
2. Knee and elbow pads.
3. Cups and supporters for males.
4. Hip and thigh pads especially for women.
5. Full finger gloves to protect fingers.
6. Education of players concerning the rules to help with safety.

Warm Up Drills

1. **Offense.**
   a. Throwing at target without blindfold.
   b. Throwing for distance from 10 to 60 feet.
   c. Practice various cues, passing ball to person giving cues.
   d. Practice all above with blindfold on.
2. **Defense.**
   a. Lunge
      1) Practice appropriate prone extension without blindfold.
      2) Practice lunging at moving ball.
      3) Practice appropriate prone extension with blindfold.
      4) Practice lunging at slow pitched ball.
      5) Increase speed of pitch and distance thrown.
      6) Practice throws from cross court and different types of throws.
   b. Auditory
      1) Practice with blindfold off, listen as ball approaches.
      2) Practice with blindfold on, throwing the ball slow at first, making sure athletes are moving in the right direction.
      3) Speed up as players improve.
   c. Connect skills by having players practice 1, 2 or 3 players at a time both offense and defense.
   d. Players need to be in constant communication with each other. They need to pay attention to how many throws in a row a player has (the maximum is 2). Have a lead person on the court.
4. **Game Drills.**
   a. Using a beach ball, have athletes throw the ball at a target. Start at 10 feet and work back to 60 feet.
   b. Same drill as above, only use a large rubber ball.
   c. Throw beach ball/rubber ball at goal area from 10 to 60 feet and different locations.

d. Practice basic lunge: begin with squat position, lunge to the right or the left. Make sure body is in prone position and fully extended. Have athletes slide into the lunge to avoid bruising the hips.

e. Lunge while trying to stop the beach ball/rubber ball. Vary the speed and direction (assistants throw the ball).

f. Have the players track the ball by listening. Have them tell assistants where it is.

g. Introduce various signals (verbal, finger-snapping, tapping on floor). Have players practice giving signals and have other players point to where the signal is coming from.

h. Have players in position on the court. Give one player the ball and have another player give a signal to pass the ball. The player with the ball tries to pass to the players giving the signal. Repeat with each player getting a chance to give signal and receive passes.

i. Put players into lanes. Player A will throw the ball to try and score on Player B. Player B will lunge to stop the ball. Player B recovers the ball and throws the ball trying to score. Start 20 feet apart and use easy throws. Increase the distance to 60 feet. Switch players. Use a large rubber ball (regulation as stated in the rules).

j. Place players in various positions on the court. Have them feel lines around them. Tell them what part of the court they are on. Switch positions until each player has been in all three positions.

k. Switching positions, have players tell assistants where they are on the court.

l. Set players up for two-on-two play.

m. Team A will throw the ball to try and score on Team B. Team B will lunge to stop the ball. Team B will recover the ball and throw it to score. Start 40 feet apart and use easy throws. Increase the distance to 60 feet. Switch teams. Practice drill with goalball.

n. Mini two-on-two tournament using goalball.

o. Practice three-person offense using passing and orientation.

p. Practice three-person defense with the assistant throwing the ball.

q. Play three-on-three scrimmage. Switch players to different positions and teams.

r. Play best two out of three games with regulation rules.

Study Questions / Learning Activities

1. Borrow a sports wheelchair and with a partner as a spotter, practice stroke and mobility techniques (including turning, cutting, ascending and descending ramps).

2. Identify the main components of a sports wheelchair.

3. Contact the National Wheelchair Athletic Association to locate any organized sporting event in your county such as track and field or basketball. Attend the event and note differences in sport wheelchairs and stroke techniques used by the various athletes. Does the stroke vary with the level of spinal cord injury (cervical versus thoracic injuries)? Explain.

References

Cooper, R. (1988). Racing chair lingo ... or how to order a racing wheelchair. *Sport N' Spokes*, March/April, 29-32.

Sherrill, C. (1986). *Adapted physical education and recreation*. Dubuque: Wm. C. Brown.

CHAPTER **15**

Emergency Procedures

The outline below designates responsibilities to a team of assistants which facilitates efficient and orderly conduct during an emergency. The procedures are designed to stabilize the injured person until advance medical personnel arrives. The procedure should be established and practiced prior to the start of the exercise program. Emergency drills should be practiced several times during the course of the program. It is suggested that each room of the facility have its own emergency team, as well as the procedures and assignments posted on a bulletin board (in full view of participants and assistants). First aid and CPR manuals and posters should be available in every room of facility, as well as an updated and replenished first aid kit in an accessible and visible location. Remember to keep detailed records of any injuries, witness accounts, and related meetings. Maintain records on insurance coverage for staff and activities in files.

Assign a Qualified Assistant to Each Specific Emergency Assignment Listed Below

1. **Begin cardiopulmonary resuscitation (CPR)/first aid.**
   a. Evaluate the victim and begin CPR as needed.
   b. Take over initial effort to revive the victim if a non-designated person is first to reach the victim.
2. **Assist with CPR — begin two-man CPR.**
3. **Call paramedics.**
   a. Every assistant in the program should be familiar with the emergency telephone procedure. However, only one assistant per class should be assigned to make the call. In most cities dialing 911 will reach an emergency dispatcher.

    b. The following information should be provided:
        1) Name and telephone number of person calling.
        2) Description of the emergency.
        3) Exact location of the emergency (have directions written before-hand).

4. **Pull the medical file.**
An assistant should have the medical file available when the paramedics arrive. This file will alert paramedics to the type of disability and the types of medication the injured person is taking. Family phone numbers, emergency contact phone number, and physicians' names and phone numbers should also be located in this file if needed.

5. **Evacuate all uninvolved individuals from the room (in the case of a serious emergency).**

6. **Assist the CPR team as a (stand-by).**
Remain by the resuscitation/first aid team in case any additional assistance, equipment, or supplies are needed.

7. **Parking lot stand-by.**
Stand in the parking lot and guide paramedics to the room where the victim is located.

First Aid

It is not within the scope of this manual to provide procedures for first aid, artificial respiration or cardiopulmonary resuscitation. Rather, it is suggested that the program director, instructors and at least two assistants (per class) obtain certification in basic first aid and cardiopulmonary resuscitation. Check your local American Red Cross for a schedule of certification classes.

Specific Emergency Procedures

For emergency procedures for specific disabilities, see Chapter 13 under:

Asthma — Emergency Procedures for an Asthma Attack (page 184).
Epilepsy — First Aid for a Tonic-Clonic Seizure (page 194).
Diabetes — Diabetic Reactions and Treatment (page 190).
Spinal Cord Injury — First Aid for Autonomic Dysreflexia (page 207).

Contraindications to Exercise Testing

It is recommended that the instructor carefully review the medical history of a participant to determine the safety of conducting a submaximal graded exercise test. Possible contraindications to testing include: (American College of Sportsmedicine, 1983)

1. Unstable angina or angina pectoris at rest.
2. Acute infectious diseases.
3. Thrombophlebitis.
4. Arrhythmias.
5. History suggesting excessive medication (i.e., digitalis, psychtropics, diuretics).
6. Untreated severe systematic or pulmonary hypertension.
7. Uncontrolled metabolic diseases (e.g., diabetes).
8. Resting blood pressure exceeding 140/90.

Indications for Termination of an Exercise or a Graded Exercise Test

Abnormal distress during exercise may indicate underlying pathology which may require further medical evaluation. The presence of the following symptoms during any exercise or graded exercise test necessitates discontinuing the activity until further medical consultation/evaluation has been obtained. These indications have been provided by the American College of Sportsmedicine (1983).

Signs and Symptoms of Exercise Intolerance

1. Dizziness or near syncope.
2. Pain or pressure in the chest, arm or throat (angina); this may be immediate or delayed.
3. Nausea or vomiting.
4. Severe fatigue; prolonged fatigue after 24 hours.
5. Severe claudication or other pain in the lower extremities.
6. Mental confusion; glassy stare.
7. Sudden lack of coordination; unsteadiness.
8. General pallor, cold sweat; blueness.
9. Lack of rapid erythematous return of skin color after brief firm compression.

Abnormal Blood Pressure Responses

1. Systolic blood pressure does not rise with increasing intensity of the exercise.
2. A drop of 10 mm Hg or more in diastolic blood pressure with successive recordings.
3. An increase in systolic blood pressure of greater than 250 mm Hg.
4. A rise in diastolic blood pressure of greater than 120 mm Hg. It is recommended by the authors that a graded exercise test (even submaximal) **not** be conducted on a person with a resting diastolic blood pressure greater than 110 mm Hg.

Abnormal Heart Rate Responses

1. A heart rate exceeding 100% of predicted (age-adjusted) maximum heart rate (standard deviation = 10 beats/minute).
2. Sudden rapid or irregular heartbeats; sudden slow pulse.
3. Poor chronotropic response.

Respiratory Responses

1. Marked dyspnea.
2. Assistance of the accessory neck and shoulder muscles for respiration (exception: spinal cord injury).

Miscellaneous Responses

The remaining symptoms listed below usually do not require any medical attention and may be remedied by some modification of the exercise program.

1. **Excessively high recovery heart rate** (i.e., heart rate remaining near target level 5 to 10 minutes after cessation of exercise).
   Remedy: Select an exercise intensity at the lower end of the target zone (e.g., 60% of predicted maximum).
2. **Dyspnea** lasting more than 10 minutes after cessation of exercise.
   Remedy: Same as #1. Make sure it is possible to carry on a conversation during exercise.
3. **Prolonged fatigue/soreness**, even 24 hours later.
   Remedy: Reduce intensity of the exercise (e.g., workload, weight to be lifted, amount of stretch achieved).
4. **Pain on the front or sides of the lower leg** (shin splints).
   Remedy: Reevaluate type of shoes worn during exercise. Swim or use stationary cycle instead of jogging. Exercise on surface which absorbs more shock.
5. **Insomnia** which was not present prior to participation in the exercise program.
   Remedy: Reduce the intensity of duration of the exercise program.
6. **Diaphragm spasm** (side stitch). Pain around lower rib cage.
   Remedy: Lean forward while sitting or standing.
7. **Muscle cramps due to over-exertion.**
   Remedy: Place muscle on stretch and hold until cramp subsides.

Medications

If a participant is taking medications, the following information should be recorded in his/her medical file for each drug: (1) name of drug, (2) purpose, (3) dose, and (4) side effects. Include medications that are taken on an infrequent or as needed basis. This information should be readily accessible in case of an emergency. Encourage the participant to become knowledgeable about the effects of medication on exercise performance. In addition, inform the assistant of any side effects which may affect the participant's exercise performance (e.g., beta- blockers may keep the heart rate depressed during aerobic exercise) or affect behavior (e.g., seizure medication such as phenobarbital may induce drowsiness). Supervision is warranted when a participant uses equipment that may be dangerous if he/she is drowsy or uncoordinated due to medication. The appearance of side effects varies among individuals and depends upon dose, individual body chemistry, and if other medications are being taken concomitantly. The side effects associated with anticonvulsant drugs are typically mild and occur only at the beginning of therapy (Epilepsy Society, 1981). In addition to prescription drugs, over-the-counter medications (e.g., colds, allergies) have side effects which may affect behavior.

Common medications and their purposes are listed below (Larson & Snobl, 1978):

1. **Urinary Tract Antibiotics** — Macrodantin, Gantrisin, Geocillin, Keflex, Septra, Ampicillin, Tetracycline.
2. **Urinary Acidifiers** — Ascorbic acid (Vitamin C) and Mandelamine are used together to acidify and sterilize the urine.
3. **Spasticity** — Valium (CNS depressant), Dantrium, Lioresal.
4. **Pain** — Aspirin, Darvon, Dolene, Tylenol.
5. **Seizures** — Dilantin, Phenobarbital, Mysoline, Tegretol, Mebaral, Diamox, Depakene.
6. **Laxatives** — Modane, Dulcolax.
7. **Stool Softeners** — Colace, Surfax.
8. **Anti-histamines** — Brompheniramine, Chlorpheniramine, Diphenhydramine, Triprolidine, Promethazine
9. **Muscle relaxant, relief of anxiety** — Diazepam

Study Questions / Learning Activities

1. Every APE program should have a posted emergency procedure with specific responsibilities assigned to qualified assistants. Create a document that describes the emergency procedure and assignments for your specific program, using the guidelines provided at the beginning of this chapter. Review this document with your instructor and compare it against the ones developed by your instructor and other assistants. Once a document has been adopted for the APE program, meet with other assistants to conduct practice drills.

2. Outline and describe first aid procedures for the following specific emergencies (see Chapter 13):

   * asthma attack
   * epileptic seizure
   * insulin reaction (diabetes)
   * autonomic dysreflexia (spinal cord injury).

3. Identify four abnormal blood pressure responses that would result in an immediate termination of exercising for a participant of any age.

4. Contact local agencies (e.g., Epilepsy Foundation, American Lung Association, Juvenile Diabetes Foundation) and have a representative visit your facility and present a lecture on first aid procedures for specific disabilities (e.g., epileptic seizure, asthma attack, diabetic reactions). These agencies may also loan videos to your program covering first aid procedures.

References

American College of Sportsmedicine (1983). *Reference guide for workshop/ certification programs in preventive/rehabilitative exercise.*

Bleck, E. E., & Nagel, D. A. (1975). *Physically handicapped children - A medical atlas for teachers.* New York: Grune & Stratton.

Epilepsy Society (1981). *Epilepsy handbook for teachers and nurses.* 1612 30th Street, San Diego, CA, 92102.

Fox, S. M., Naughton, S. P., & Haskell, W. L. (1971). Physical activity and the prevention of coronary heart disease. *Annuals of Clinical Research, 3,* 404.

Larson, M. R. & Snobl, D. E. (1978). *Attendant care manual.* Minnesota: Rehabilitation Service, Southwest State University.

APPENDIX

Abbreviations

The following abbreviations are typically found on medical histories, physical evaluations, prescriptions and exercise programs for persons with disabilities. This acceptable format expedites the process of filling in forms and results in consistency among personnel. Some of the abbreviations have been created by the authors and found to be useful in writing exercise programs. The instructor and assistants should become familiar with these abbreviations and their meanings.

@	at	<	less than
ADL	Activities of Daily Living	LE	lower extremity
AK	Above knee	LOM	limitation of motion
AMA	against medical advice	L-S Spine	lumbosacral spine
ant.	anterior	MBC	maximum breathing capacity
A.P.	anterior-posterior	meds	medications
b.i.d.	twice a day	mg	milligram
BK	Below knee	M.I.	myocardial infarction
B.M.R.	Basal metabolic rate	>	more than
BP	blood presure		
bpm	beats per minute	ō	none
		O₂	oxygen
c̄	with	Op	operation
CCU	Coronary Care Unit	O.T.	Occupational Therapy
cm	centimeter		
CNS	Central nervous system	p̄	after
C/O	complains of	‖ bars	parallel bars
CPR	cardiopulmonary resuscitation	Post-op	post-operative
C-Spine	cervical spine	PRE	Progressive Resistive Exercise
CVA	cerebrovascular accident	pt.	patient
Δ	change in	P.T.	Physical Therapy
D.C.	discontinue	PVC	premature ventricular contraction
disch.	discharge	PWB	partial weight bearing
DOE	dyspnea on exertion	q.d.	every day or daily
Dx	diagnosis	q.h.	every hour
	decrease	RHR	resting heart rate
E.C.G.	electrocardiogram	ROM	range of motion
E.E.G.	electroencephalogram	rpm	revolutions per minute
E.M.G.	electromyogram	® or Rt.	right
etiol.	etiology	Rx	prescription
F.B.S.	fasting blood sugar	-	
FWB	full weight bearing	s̄	without
Fx	fracture	SCI	spinal cord injury
gm	gram	2°	secondary to
ht.	height	SOB	shortness of breath
Hx	history	THR	target heart rate
I.C.U.	Intensive Care Unit	t.i.d.	three times per day
I.E.P.	Individualized Education Program	V.A.	Veteran's Administration
	increase	V.C.	Vital Capacity
I.V.	intravenous	WNL	within normal limits
L or Lt.	left	wt.	weight
LBP	low back pain	x	times

B

Diagram of Court for Goalball

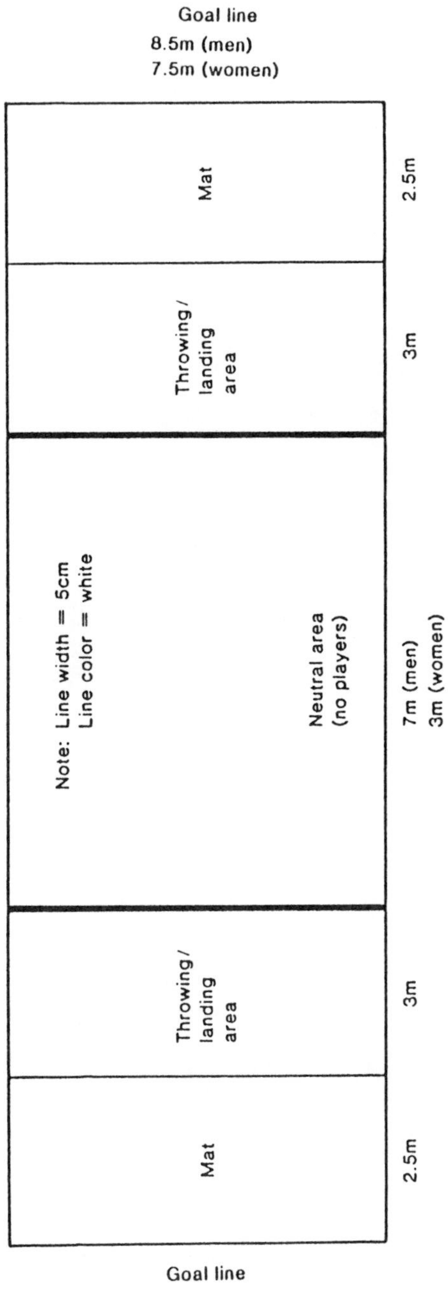

Goal line
8.5m (men)
7.5m (women)

Mat — 2.5m

Throwing / landing area — 3m

Note: Line width = 5cm
Line color = white

Neutral area (no players) — 7m (men) / 3m (women)

Throwing / landing area — 3m

Mat — 2.5m

Goal line

Posture Grid

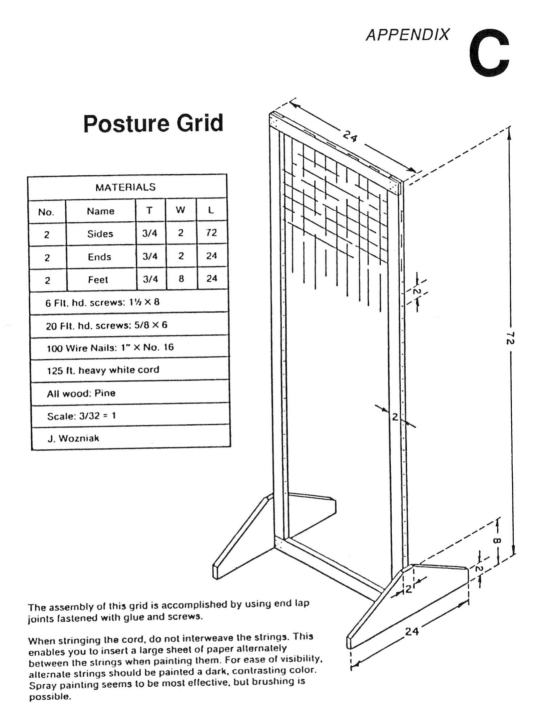

MATERIALS				
No.	Name	T	W	L
2	Sides	3/4	2	72
2	Ends	3/4	2	24
2	Feet	3/4	8	24

6 Flt. hd. screws: 1½ × 8

20 Flt. hd. screws: 5/8 × 6

100 Wire Nails: 1" × No. 16

125 ft. heavy white cord

All wood: Pine

Scale: 3/32 = 1

J. Wozniak

The assembly of this grid is accomplished by using end lap joints fastened with glue and screws.

When stringing the cord, do not interweave the strings. This enables you to insert a large sheet of paper alternately between the strings when painting them. For ease of visibility, alternate strings should be painted a dark, contrasting color. Spray painting seems to be most effective, but brushing is possible.

(Photo courtesy of J. Wozniak, LaCrosse, Wis.).

D

Sit-And-Reach Apparatus

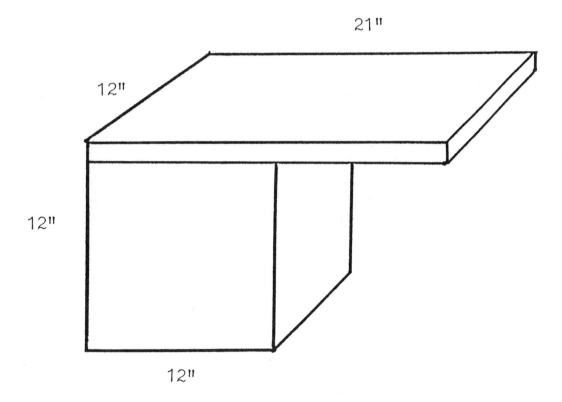

Quad Gloves

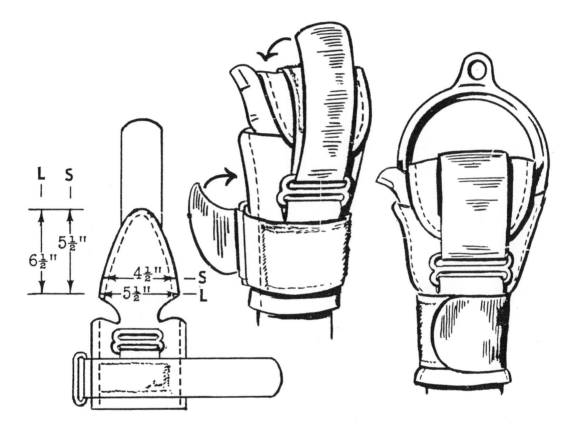

Anecdotal Record for the Participant with Epilepsy

What did the student do before the seizure (precipitating events, if any)?

_____

_____

What did the student do during the seizure (sides and parts of the body most affected during the seizure)?

_____

_____

How did the student act after the seizure?_____

_____

Duration of seizure: _____   Time of day:_____

Reaction of other students: _____

_____

_____

Any injuries sustained as a result of the seizure? _____

_____

Does the student exhibit any unusual activity that could be a resulting side effect of anticonvulsant medication (drowsiness, inattention, irritability, etc.)?

_____

_____

Additional comments: *(This area should be used for answering questions listed under* "Observing the Seizure.")

*   *This kind of record should be kept with the knowledge and written consent of student and parents, and should be sent to parents or physician after each seizure.*

Glossary

The following section is a simple dictionary containing a list of terms frequently used in APE programs. The short definition of these words should be of help to instructors and assistants when reading medical reports, attending medically-related meetings, and talking with other specialists who are involved with the participant.

Achilles Flare
: A bowing of the Achilles tendon toward the midline (Helbing's sign) which is associated with eversion or pronation of the foot.

Activities of Daily Living
: Self-care activities performed on a daily basis in order to maintain health and well-being (e.g. getting in and out of bed, personal hygiene, eating, performing manual tasks, ambulating or using a wheelchair).

Adam's Position
: From a standing position with the feet together, flex forward at the hips while allowing the trunk to relax, head down, and arms to hang down with the palms together. Used to determine structural scoliosis.

Adaptive Behavior
: Behavior that aids the individual in effective, age-appropriate social interactions, mobility, and independence.

Afferent
: Carrying impulses to a center (input) such as the central nervous system. Refers to sensory neurons.

Affective
: Pertains to feelings or emotions.

Amputation
: Congenital or acquired loss of an extremity or portion thereof.

Anomalies
: Congenital deformity or abnormal development of organ, tissue or bone.

Aphasia
: An inability to interpret or execute spoken language (receptive and expressive, respectively) which is not related to diseases of the vocal cords or ears.

Apraxia
: Inability to motor plan (i.e., execute a series of movements in a coordinated and efficient manner). Probably related to poor input from the tactile, vestibular and proprioceptive systems.

Arteriosclerosis	Thickening or hardening of the walls of the blood vessels, particularly the arteries.
Articular	The area of a bone where it is joined together with another bone as a joint.
Ataxia	Difficulties with balance; reflected in a gait pattern that utilizes by a wide base of support. A type of cerebral palsy in which balance is affected. Generally involves a medical condition of the cerebellum.
Atherosclerosis	A build up of plaque in the arteries.
Athetosis	A type of cerebral palsy which is characterized by rotary, involuntary movements Involves a medical condition of the basal ganglia.
Auditory Discrimination	The ability to detect subtle differences among sounds in words (e.g., tap-cap, then-than).
Behavior Modification	A procedure that is based on the assumption that all behaviors are learned and depend upon consequences. Therefore, behavior can be changed through a methodically applied system of rewards and punishments.
Behavioral Objectives	Objectives which are written to describe what a student will be able to do as a result of some planned instruction. These are usually written as objectives that can be measured in some definitive or quantitative way.
Bilateral Coordination	A lack of coordination between the two sides of the body. An inability to use the two hands and/or legs together in a coordinated fashion. If unable to cross the midline of the body, the individual may appear ambidextrous (using the left hand on the left side only and vice-versa)
Body Awareness	The ability to locate and identify body parts. Also includes an awareness of the relationship of the body parts to each other and to the environment. The development of the body scheme is based on receiving accurate sensory information from the skin, muscles, and joints (i.e., proprioception).
Brain Stem	Consists of the medulla, pons, and midbrain.
Cardiac	Pertaining to the heart.

Catheter	A tube used for evacuating fluid from the bladder or brain. In the case of the bladder, the catheter may be in-dwelling or external.
Cauda Equina	The terminal portion of the spinal cord (conus medullaris) and roots of the spinal nerves below the first lumbar nerve.
Central Nervous System	Consists of the spinal cord, brain stem, cerebellum, and cerebrum.
Contraindicated	Not advised. Used often in reference to an exercise that should not be performed because of a particular medical condition of an individual.
Coordination, Fine Motor	Pertains to usage of small muscle groups for manipulation (e.g., writing, cutting).
Coordination, Gross Motor	Pertains to usage of large muscle groups for locomotion and manipulation (e.g., jumping, running, throwing, catching).
Diplegia	Paralysis/paresis of all four extremities, with more severe involvement of the lower extremities.
Directionality	The ability to determine directions and locations in the environment (e.g., left, right, up, down, over, under, across, through). The concept of moving right or left.
Dysfunction	Difficult function, improper function, or non-function.
Efferent	Carrying impulses away from a center (output) such as the central nervous system. Refers to motoneurons.
Equilibrium Reactions (Cortical)	The automatic movements which keep one balanced during static and dynamic postures such as sitting, standing, and walking. Involves automatic responses of the head, trunk and limbs.
Etiology	The cause of a medical condition.
Grand Mal (Tonic-Clonic) Seizure	One of the more serious forms of epilepsy which involves stiffening and convulsions of the body.
Habilitation	Maximizing the potential of an individual who is disabled from birth.
Hemiplegia	Paralysis of one side of the body.

Intelligence Tests	A standardized series of questions and/or tasks designed to measure mental abilities (i.e., how a person thinks, reasons, solves problems, remembers, and learns new information). Many intelligence tests rely heavily on the use or understanding of spoken language.
Kinesthesis	The ability to perceive the position or movement of body parts and the amount of force exerted by the muscles.
Laterality	The awareness of the sides of the body — right, left, front, back, side, top, bottom.
Lordosis	Hyperextension of the lumbar spine.
Lumbar	The area of the low back.
Monoplegia	Paralysis of one extremity only.
Muscle Substitution	The employment of a different muscle or muscle group to replace a muscle that can no longer be used.
Paralysis	Lack of innervation to muscle, resulting in loss of voluntary motion.
Paresis	Muscular weakness.
Paraplegia	Paralysis of the lower extremities only.
Perseveration	Inability to stop responding to a stimulus or a directive.
Pronation	Eversion combined with abduction of the foot.
Prone	Lying in a face-down position.
Proprioception	Sensory feedback concerning movement and position of the body, occurring chiefly in the muscles (spindles), tendons (Golgi tendon organs), and joint receptors.
Psychomotor	Pertaining to movement (both fine and gross motor).
Pulmonary	Pertaining to lung function, heart valve function, or the pulmonary artery.
Quadriplegia	Paralysis affecting all four limbs.
Range of Motion	Degree of movement possible about a joint.

Scoliosis	An abnormal lateral curvature in any region of the spine.
Seizure	Abnormal electrical output of the brain.
Sensory Integration	Neurological process of organizing information from one or more sensory channel.
Spasticity	A neurological disorder of the upper motoneuron, resulting in abnormally active stretch reflexes. Muscle appears hypertonic and demonstrates exaggerated reflexes or clonus when perturbed (i.e., stretched).
Spatial Awareness/Orientation	The awareness of one's position in space and the location of objects in relation to self and other objects. Includes judgements of distance, depth and directionality.
Tactile	Pertaining to the sense of touch; discrimination of texture and shape; detection of pressure, heat, and pain.